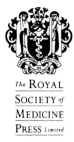

The ROYAL
SOCIETY *of*
MEDICINE
PRESS *Limited*

Rheumatoid
Arthritis

in Practice

Peter C Taylor

BA (Oxon) MA (Cantab) BM BCh PhD FRCP
Professor of Experimental Rheumatology and
Head of Clinical Trials, The Kennedy Institute
of Rheumatology Division, Imperial College
London, UK and Honorary Consultant
Physician and Rheumatologist, Charing Cross
Hospital, London, UK

© 2007 Royal Society of Medicine Press Ltd

Reprinted 2007

Published by the Royal Society of Medicine Press Ltd
1 Wimpole Street, London W1G 0AE, UK
Tel: +44 (0) 20 7290 2921
Fax: +44 (0) 20 7290 2929
Email: publishing@rsm.ac.uk
Website: www.rsmpress.co.uk

British Library Cataloguing in Publication Data

A catalogue record for this book is available from the British Library

ISBN ISBN 1-85315-670-1
ISSN 1473-6845

Distribution in Europe and Rest of World:
Marston Book Services Ltd
PO Box 269
Abingdon
Oxon OX14 4YN, UK
Tel: +44 (0) 1235 465 500
Fax: +44 (0) 1235 465 555
Email: direct.order@marston.com

Distribution in Australia and New Zealand:
Elsevier Australia
30–52 Smidmore Street
Marrickville NSW 2204
Australia
Tel: + 61 2 9517 8999
Fax: + 61 2 9517 2249
Email: service@elsevier.com.au

Distribution in the USA and Canada:
Royal Society of Medicine Press Ltd
c/o BookMasters, Inc.
30 Amberwood Parkway
Ashland, OH 44805, USA
Tel: +1 800 247 6553 / +1 800 266 5564
Fax: +1 419 281 6883
E-mail: order@bookmasters.com

Typeset by Phoenix Photosetting, Chatham, Kent, UK
Printed in Great Britain by Marston Book Services Limited, Oxford

About the author

Dr Peter C Taylor is Professor of Experimental Rheumatology and Head of the Clinical Trials Group at the Kennedy Institute of Rheumatology Division, Imperial College, London. He studied preclinical medical sciences at Gonville and Caius College at the University of Cambridge and his first degree was in Physiology. He subsequently studied clinical medicine at the University of Oxford and was awarded a PhD degree from the University of London for studies on pathogenesis of arthritis.

Dr Taylor has specialist clinical interests in rheumatoid arthritis and early inflammatory arthritis. His research interests are in the use of novel imaging for evaluation of prognosis, the assessment of responses to therapy and as an early indicator of disease modification, as well as mechanisms sustaining inflammatory joint disease. Over the last 10 years, he has been a principal investigator in numerous clinical trials of biological therapies for rheumatoid arthritis and mechanism of action studies employing anti-cytokine therapy as probes of pathogenesis. He is a Faculty Member of the Innovative Therapies & Advances in Standard Therapies Evaluation Board, Faculty of 1000 Medicine.

Acknowledgements

I would like to express my gratitude to Meg James for her skilled secretarial assistance in preparation of the text.

Contents

Introduction

Rheumatoid arthritis is the commonest form of inflammatory arthritis. It affects approximately 1% of the population in the Western world and is, therefore, a condition familiar to most physicians. Untreated, or sub-optimally treated, it generally becomes progressively disabling over time causing significant suffering for patients as well as their families and friends. Despite this, there has been a dramatic improvement in the outlook for most patients over the last decade. This has, in part, been a consequence of the growing appreciation of the gravity of the social and economic burden imposed by this condition as well as the increased co-morbidity and mortality associated with inadequate suppression of inflammation over time. The improved outlook has come about in a number of ways. First, there have been very considerable advances in the treatment options for rheumatoid arthritis, most notably with the introduction of new classes of effective biological (protein-based, parenterally administered) therapies directed against key pathogenic targets. Although the primary cause of rheumatoid arthritis remains unknown, this has been possible because of advances in molecular technology that have facilitated identification of novel therapeutic targets including cell subsets, cytokines, and other molecules that contribute to the inflammatory and destructive components of the disease. Concurrent advances in biotechnology have permitted production of abundant, high-quality monoclonal antibodies or fusion proteins, suitable for administration to patients, which specifically bind to one of these targets. The most notable success to date has been the introduction of biological agents blocking the activity of the pro-inflammatory cytokine TNF-α. Second, management approaches have also undergone a major evolutionary change. This has come about with improved understanding of the most effective use and dosing of both conventional and biological drug treatments; in particular, that optimum outcomes are achieved when synovitis is suppressed as completely as possible. Furthermore, there is now compelling evidence that disease outcome is particularly favourable when treatment intervention is initiated as soon as possible after symptom onset.

Although major advances in treatment of rheumatoid arthritis in the last two decades have been in the field of therapeutics, the successful management of rheumatoid arthritis is not dependent on pharmacological intervention alone. Patients may require help and support from many members of a multidisciplinary team all of whom have an important role in patient education and bring different sets of expertise to bear in minimising the impact of disease and optimising joint function and overall well being.

However, rheumatoid arthritis is not yet curable. So it is important to emphasise that, although the outlook for patients with this condition is now better than it has ever been in the past, there remain numerous areas of unmet need. These include development of therapies for patients who are refractory to existing drug treatment; new therapies with superior efficacy to those currently available with benefits in a higher proportion of patients; development of more convenient routes of administration and, in particular, cheaper production costs, for example oral drugs delivering benefits as least as high as those of biological TNF inhibitors. Ideally, improved safety profiles or easy reversibility of drug-related toxicity would be desirable. Other unmet needs include the development of biomarkers that reliably inform management treatment decisions on an individual patient basis. For example, a rheumatologist needs to know which patients would most benefit from biological therapies, and how can a satisfactory response to therapy be evaluated accurately, not only in terms of how the patient feels, but also with respect to inhibition of structural damage to joints at an early stage of treatment intervention. These and other clinically relevant questions help to set the current and future clinical research agenda.

This book aims to provide an update on rheumatoid arthritis covering a broad range of relevant background including clinical disease expression, current knowledge of pathogenesis, role of the multidisciplinary team, and an overview of conventional drug therapies. Furthermore, in view of the rapid pace of development in thinking regarding the management approach to rheumatoid arthritis, recent advances in treatment are reviewed including clinical trial data for the use of biological therapies. It is hoped that this work will be of value to primary care practitioners, junior hospital doctors and those training in rheumatology as well as all those with involvement in the care of arthritic patients or working in the pharmaceutical industry with an interest in rheumatic diseases.

1 Definition and pathology

Definition
Clinical features
Differential diagnosis
Natural history and outcomes
Epidemiology

Definition

Rheumatoid arthritis is best thought of as a syndrome. In its established phase, it is generally straightforward to recognise. However, the variability of the presentation and clinical course in the early stages of the illness is such that diagnosis, or classification, can be very difficult. Whether the diagnosis is beyond doubt or uncertain, it is very important that primary care practitioners refer such patients to a secondary care specialist at the earliest possible date. This is because in recent years it has become recognised that more favourable clinical outcomes are achieved when synovitis is optimally suppressed early in the course of disease. The evidence for this and suggested criteria for referral will be discussed later.

Once established, rheumatoid arthritis is characterised by a deforming symmetrical polyarthritis of varying extent and severity. It may be associated with synovitis of joint and tendon sheaths, articular cartilage loss, erosion of juxta-articular bone and, in a majority of patients, the presence of IgM rheumatoid factor in the blood. In a proportion of patients, systemic and extra-articular features may be observed during the course of disease (and rarely prior to joint disease). Such features include anaemia, weight loss, vasculitis, serositis, nodules in subcutaneous, pulmonary, and sclera tissues, mononeuritis multiplex, and pulmonary interstitial inflammation as well as exocrine, salivary, and lachrymal gland involvement.

The clinical presentation is heterogeneous, with a wide spectrum of age of onset, degree of joint involvement, and severity. Similarly, the disease course is variable. It ranges from a brief, mild, self-limiting oligo-articular illness with minimal joint damage to a sustained polyarticular synovial inflammation resulting in relentlessly progressive cartilage destruction, erosion of bone, and ultimately changes in joint integrity, with corresponding functional impairment.

The American College of Rheumatology has developed and revised classification criteria for the diagnosis of rheumatoid arthritis, based on a hospital population of patients with established active disease. These criteria combine a constellation of clinical, serological, and radiological features, and have become widely accepted for epidemiological and clinical studies. By emphasising key features of the syndrome, the criteria help to differentiate rheumatoid arthritis from other forms of inflammatory arthritis, with a diagnostic sensitivity and specificity of about 90% for active disease. However, these requirements have a much poorer sensitivity for a diagnosis of rheumatoid arthritis in the early stages of presentation, where the sensitivity of the classification criteria ranges from 40% to 60%, and the specificity is no better than 80–90%.[1–6] There are seven components to the American College of Rheumatology classification criteria for rheumatoid arthritis (Table 1.1).[7] Rheumatoid arthritis is defined by the presence of four or more of these criteria.[7]

It will be noted that of the seven components of the American College of Rheumatology classification criteria, five are clinical. However, rheumatoid nodules are very rare in the early phase of rheumatoid arthritis. One of the remaining four clinical criteria relates to involvement of at least three joint areas whereas rheumatoid arthritis frequently first presents as a mono- or oligo-articular disease.

Table 1.1
American College of Rheumatology criteria for the classification of rheumatoid arthritis

1   Morning stiffness in and around joints for at least 1 hour
2   Soft tissue swelling of three or more joints observed by a physician
3   Swelling (arthritis) of proximal interphalangeal, metacarpophalangeal, or wrist joints
4   Symmetrical swelling of joints
5   Subcutaneous rheumatoid nodules
6   Presence of IgM rheumatoid factor in abnormal amounts
7   Radiographic erosions and/or peri-articular osteopenia in hand and/or wrist joints

Criteria 1–4 of at least 4 weeks' duration.

There is only one imaging criterion and that is based on radiographic assessment. Again, this is met only rarely in the early phase of disease. In patients with symptom duration of less than 3 months who subsequently went on to meet classification criteria for rheumatoid arthritis, erosions were found in only 13%.[2]

By 2 years after symptom onset, joint erosions are present in 50–70% of rheumatoid arthritis patients.[8] Similarly, the 1987 classification criteria include only one serological test, namely rheumatoid factor. This is seen less frequently in the early phase of disease than in established disease.[9]

In view of these considerations, there is now a need to revise classification criteria for rheumatoid arthritis, or at least to define better early prognostic factors for persistent inflammatory joint disease and structural damage to joints in order that appropriate medication can be started before any irreversible joint damage takes place.

Other useful imaging and serological tests not included in the 1987 classification criteria for rheumatoid arthritis

Antibodies to citrullinated peptides

It has long been known that anti-perinuclear factor and anti-keratin antibodies have high specificity for rheumatoid arthritis. In fact, both these antibodies recognise epidermal fillagrin, a protein involved in the cornification of the epidermis. The amino acid target of these antibodies is citrulline, which is derived from the amino acid arginine after peptide translation under the influence of the enzyme peptidyl arginine deiminase (Fig. 1.1). Antibodies directed at citrullinated peptides have a similar sensitivity to rheumatoid factor, but higher specificity.[10]

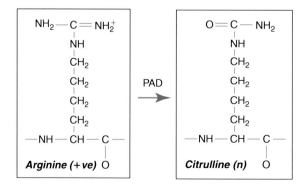

Figure 1.1
Post-translational conversion of arginine to citrulline by the enzyme peptidyl arginine deiminase (PAD).

As in the case of high-titre rheumatoid factor, antibodies to citrullinated peptides are associated with persistence and destructiveness of rheumatoid arthritis. They may also precede the onset of clinical disease.

Imaging

Synovitis is not invariably coupled to joint destruction, although this is the most serious accompaniment of inflammation, with the potential to lead to progressive loss of function. Plain radiography offers only late signs of preceding disease activity and resulting cartilage and bone destruction. Although it remains the most widely used imaging modality, it has a number of limitations. These include the use of ionising radiation and projectional superimposition that can obscure erosions and mimic cartilage loss as an inevitable consequence of presenting a three-dimensional structure in only two planes.[12] In comparison, images obtained using newer magnetic resonance and ultrasonographic technologies emphasise the inadequacy of plain radiography for soft tissue assessment in rheumatoid arthritis and can detect the presence of erosions in early disease with greater sensitivity than plain radiography (Fig. 1.2).[13,14]

At the present time there is much research interest in standardising newer imaging technologies for the assessment of rheumatoid arthritis and, in the case of MRI, in determining the pathophysiological correlates of imaging abnormalities. It is very likely that we will see increasing use of these tools in the future to inform management decisions better, suppress synovitis at an early stage optimally and improve treatment outcomes.

Clinical features

Presentation

Common patterns

Rheumatoid arthritis often begins insidiously with joint pain and stiffness, which may be associated with swelling. The joints most commonly involved first are the metacarpophalangeal joints, proximal interphalangeal joints, wrists, and metatarsophalangeal joints. There may be only

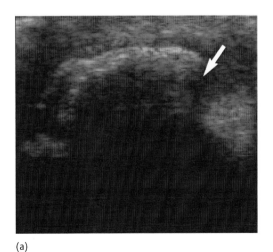
(a)

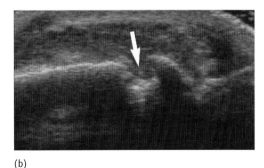
(b)

Figure 1.2
Detection of erosions by high frequency ultrasonography. (a) Transverse metacarpal–phalangeal joint; (b) longitudinal metacarpal–phalangeal joint.

a few joints involved initially (oligo-articular onset) with subsequent progression to involvement of multiple joints in a symmetrical distribution over a time period spanning weeks to months. Patients often report marked stiffness of joints on waking in the morning, and also following periods of inactivity. This stiffness may last at least an hour. There is often progressive decline in physical function with loss of grip strength and difficulty undertaking simple everyday tasks such as doing up buttons, undoing jar lids, or turning on taps. Fatigue and lethargy are also common features and there may be an accompanying low-grade fever and weight loss. Although symptoms tend to be persistent in affected joints, there may also be day-to-day variation in severity. The relapsing and remitting nature of rheumatoid arthritis, and the tendency of symptoms to move from one joint area to another, is reflected in the root of the word 'rheumatoid', which is derived from the Greek *rheum* (ρευμ) meaning 'to flow'. In most cases, however, with the passage of time more joints become involved and the distribution of arthritis becomes permanently established.

Other patterns of clinical presentation

- In up to one-third of patients, the presentation may be that of a sudden, severe, or subacute arthritis which rapidly leads to loss of function and markedly restricted mobility

- A migratory polyarthritis that 'flits' from joint to joint may be observed in a minority of patients. This presentation is referred to as 'palindromic rheumatism'. It may be a recurring pattern over many months before a more typical rheumatoid pattern becomes established and in some cases it may remit altogether

- In about 10% of cases, typically in patients over the age of 55 years, the presenting features may be indistinguishable from polymyalgia rheumatica. These comprise marked limb girdle pain and stiffness, with painful movement of the neck, shoulders, and hips

- Rheumatoid arthritis may present as a persistent inflammatory mono-arthritis and this may antedate the onset of polyarticular disease by many months or even years. Joints that can be involved include the knee, wrist, ankle, shoulder, or hip

- Other patients may present with diffuse bilateral swelling of the fingers and hands, together with symptoms and signs of carpal tunnel syndrome

- Tenosynovitis of the hands, involving the dorsal extensors of the wrist and flexor tendons in the palm and wrist, may occur at the same time as joint swelling or independently

- In rare cases, rheumatoid syndrome may present with extra-articular manifestations of disease, such as subcutaneous nodules, pleurisy with pleural effusion, pericarditis, episcleritis, or vasculitis.

Joint distribution

The most commonly involved joints during the course of rheumatoid arthritis are summarised in Table 1.2

Clinical features of joint disease

Hands and wrists

Soft tissue swelling and tenderness of the metacarpal–phalangeal and proximal interphalangeal joints accompany the active phase of disease. Flexor tendons in the palms may be palpably thickened and nodular; in some cases, this is accompanied by triggering of the fingers. Carpal tunnel syndrome may be a complication of wrist tendonitis and wrist synovitis. In established disease, wasting of the interossii is prominent and patients may not be able to make a full fist. With time, ulnar deviation and volar subluxation may develop at the metacarpophalangeal joints, with volar subluxation and radial deviation at the wrists. In addition, the ulnar styloid may become dorsally subluxed. In these later stages, the

Table 1.2
Most commonly involved joints during the course of rheumatoid arthritis

Site involved	Approximate percentage of patients with particular joints involved during course of illness
Hands	
Metacarpal–phalangeal joints	90–95%
Proximal interphalangeal joints	65–90%
Wrists	80–90%
Elbow	40–50%
Shoulder	50–60%
Hip	40–50%
Knee	60–80%
Ankle: talar joints	50–80%
Feet: metatarsal–phalangeal joints	50–90%
Cervical spine, especially C1–2	33–50%
Temporomandibular joint	20–30%

extensor tendons are stretched across the shrunken carpus so that they appear prominent in the so-called 'bowstring' sign. Tenosynovium may either be encapsulating or locally invasive, in which case there is a risk of tendon rupture. Extensor tendon rupture needs to be recognised rapidly and referred to a hand surgeon if repair is to be successful. The most commonly involved tendons are the extensor tendons of the little or ring fingers.

Digital vascular occlusive disease, particularly in long-standing rheumatoid arthritis, may result in nail fold and fingertip infarcts and splinter haemorrhages. Palmar erythema may also occur.

Common hand deformities in established rheumatoid arthritis

- Fusiform swelling – spindle-shaped distal fingers as a consequence of synovitis of proximal inter-phalangeal joints
- Boutonnière deformity – fixed flexion of the proximal interphalangeal joint and hyperextension of the distal interphalangeal joint caused by weakening of the central slip of the extrinsic extensor tendon, and a palmar displacement of the lateral bands (Fig. 1.3a)

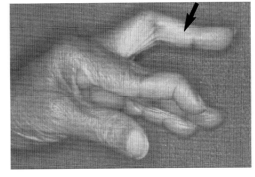
(a)

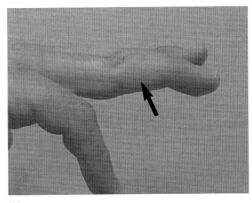
(b)

Figure 1.3
Boutonnière (a) and swan-neck (b) deformities.

- Swan-neck deformity – fixed flexion of the distal interphalangeal joint, hyperextension of the proximal interphalangeal joint, and flexion contracture of the metacarpophalangeal joint resulting from contraction of the flexors (Fig. 1.3b)
- Piano-key ulnar head – secondary to the destruction of the ulnar collateral ligament.

Feet and ankles

Involvement of the metatarsophalangeal joints is common, leading to subluxation of the metatarsal heads and eventually to claw or hammer-toe deformities. The consequence of this is that patients have problems fitting their toes into shoes, as the tops of the toes rub against the shoe material, resulting in callus or ulcer formation. Furthermore, as the soft tissue pad that normally resides beneath the metatarsal heads is displaced, the heads of the metatarsal bones are effectively exposed and no longer cushioned. As a result, walking becomes painful and patients often complain that they feel as if they are walking on pebbles.

Flattening of the arches of the foot and hind-foot valgus deformity may occur as a result of arthritic involvement of the tarsal joint and subtalar joint. This, in turn, can cause callosities where hind-foot abnormalities rub against poorly fitting shoes, and emphasises the importance of comfortable footwear in the management of rheumatoid arthritis.

Elbows and shoulders

Where these joints are involved, in the early stages common symptoms include pain and limitation of movement. The elbow may become swollen and olecranon bursitis is common. The extensor surface of the elbow is a common site for subcutaneous nodules. Pronation and supernation of the elbow may become restricted and, in time, involvement of the head of the proximal radial ulnar joints may lead to dislocation. At the shoulder, sub-acromial bursitis may result in a painful arc, and there may be involvement of the rotator cuff and biceps tendons.

Knees and hips

The knees are commonly involved and joint destruction can result in marked deterioration in mobility. Weakening of the joint capsule is such that when pressure in the knee joint is raised during active flexion, the joint can rupture with leakage of inflammatory fluid into the calf, with consequent swelling and pain resembling a deep vein thrombosis. Chronic accumulation of fluid in the knee joint may be associated with a palpable posterior popliteal (Baker's) cyst, which can increase in size on walking.

Hips are less commonly involved than knees, although secondary degenerative disease of the hips can occur. In severe rheumatoid involvement of the hip joints, there may be re-modelling of the outer acetabulum, resulting in protrusio acetabuli.

Cervical spine involvement

Between a third and a half of rheumatoid arthritis patients have involvement of the cervical spine, most commonly at the C1–2 levels. Subluxation may cause pain radiating to the occiput and, if there is instability, it may impinge on the spinal cord. It is, therefore, important to recognise this condition as sudden death may occur. It is particularly important to obtain radiographic views of the cervical spine prior to undertaking any surgical procedure that requires intubation.

The most common pattern of cervical spine involvement is atlanto-axial subluxation, which accounts for about half of the cases seen. The most frequent pattern is anterior subluxation caused by synovitis around the articulation of the odontoid process, with the anterior arch of C1, with subsequent stretching and rupture of the transverse and alar ligaments. This is detected radiographically as a gap of greater than 3 mm between the arch of C1 and the odontoid peg. When the anterior atlanto-odontoid interval exceeds 9 mm, there is very high risk of spinal cord compression.

- Much more rarely, collapse of the lateral articulations between C1 and C2 results in vertical atlanto-axial subluxation such that the odontoid peg impinges on the brainstem; this has a poor prognosis
- About a third of patients with cervical spine involvement have C1–2 impaction with destruction between the occipito-atlantal and atlanto-axial joint
- In about 15% of the patients with cervical spine involvement it is at a subaxial level, most commonly of the C2–3 and C3–4 facets and introvertible discs. This can lead to spondylovasesis, with one vertebra subluxing forward on the lower vertebra.

Extra-articular disease

Although rheumatoid arthritis has its principal manifestation in joints, it is in fact a chronic systemic inflammatory condition in which a wide variety of extra-articular features may develop (Fig, 1.4; Table 1.3). These occur predominantly in patients who are rheumatoid factor positive and carry the HLA-DR4 gene. Furthermore, extra-articular features are more likely to occur in male patients. Some of the systemic features of rheumatoid arthritis may mimic those occurring with co-morbid conditions, for example, cachexia and low-grade fever; therefore, it is important to exclude malignancy, infection, or other co-morbid causes before concluding that the systemic features are part of the rheumatoid syndrome, particularly in patients who are seronegative for rheumatoid factor.

Rheumatoid nodules

Rheumatoid nodules occur in about 20–35% of rheumatoid arthritis patients. These patients are typically seropositive for rheumatoid factor and have severe disease. Rheumatoid nodules are subcutaneous and have a characteristic histological picture, with a central area of fibrinoid necrosis surrounded by a zone of palisading elongating histiocytes and a peripheral layer of cellular connective tissue. They typically occur on the extensor surface of

Table 1.3
Extra-articular manifestations of rheumatoid arthritis

General	Cardiac
Fever	Pericarditis
Lymphadenopathy	Myocarditis
Weight loss	Coronary vasculitis
Fatigue	Nodules on valves
Dermatological	*Ocular*
Erythema	Episcleritis
Subcutaneous nodules	Scleritis
Vasculitis	Choroid and retinal nodules
Pulmonary	*Haematological*
Pleuritis	Felty's syndrome
Nodules	Large granular lymphocyte
Interstitial lung disease	syndrome
Bronchiolitis obliterans	Lymphomas
Arteritis	
Neuromuscular	*Exocrine gland involvement*
Entrapment neuropathy	Sjøgren's syndrome
Peripheral neuropathy	
Mononeuritis multiplex	
Other	
Secondary amyloidosis	

the forearms, in the olecranon bursa, over joints, and over pressure points, for example, the ischial tuberosity or heel. They may also occur on the dorsum of the fingers and methotrexate therapy is associated with nodulosis in the form of multiple small rapidly-evolving nodules which can appear even when the disease is otherwise well controlled.

Ocular manifestations of rheumatoid arthritis

Episcleritis and scleritis are within the spectrum of extra-articular manifestations. If scleral inflammation is persistent, scleral thinning can occur, with a risk of complicating scleromalacia perforans. These complications require specialist review and treatment by an ophthalmologist. Keratoconjunctivitis sicca frequently accompanies concomitant secondary Sjøgren's syndrome.

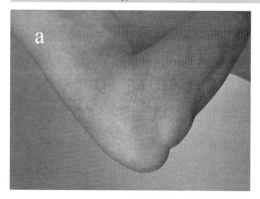

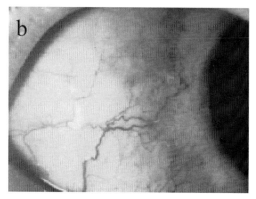

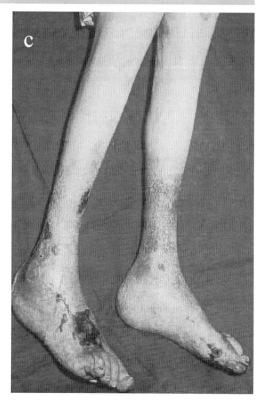

Figure 1.4
Some extra-articular features of rheumatoid arthritis. (a) Nodules at the elbow; (b) scleritis; and (c) vasculitis.

Pulmonary manifestations

Pleurisy and pleural effusions can complicate rheumatoid arthritis, and, rarely, may be the presenting feature. Pleural aspirates confirm the effusion to be a cellular exudate enriched in lymphocytes but also containing polymorphonuclear cells and macrophages. There are high protein concentrations and lactate dehydrogenase levels, but low glucose, usually than 1.4 mmol/l, because of a defect in transportation of glucose across the pleura.

Rheumatoid nodules can occur in the lung as solitary or multiple masses. They tend to be peripheral and may cavitate or even spontaneously resolve. A less commonly seen variant these days can occur in patients whose occupation was in the coal mining industry, when multiple rheumatoid nodules can occur. This is known as Caplan's syndrome. Pulmonary function testing in established rheumatoid arthritis often reveals abnormalities suggestive of airways and interstitial disease, even in the absence of any symptoms. Fibrosing alveolitis is only symptomatic and progressive in fewer than 10% of patients, however. This occurs more frequently in male than female patients. They are usually seropositive and have a high frequency of anti-nuclear antibodies, with other features of multisystem disease.

Obliterative bronchiolitis usually presents with a rapidly progressive dyspnoea. A chest radiograph reveals hyper-inflated lungs and pulmonary function tests show small airways obstruction. The condition can be rapidly fatal but other patients follow a more chronic protracted course that may respond to corticosteroid and immunosuppressive therapy. In the past, when penicillamine was used more widely, this was occasionally associated with obliterative bronchiolitis. Obliterative bronchiolitis can also be associated with organising pneumonia (Boop) and may respond to corticosteroid therapy. A non-specific interstitial pneumonitis responsive to corticosteroids may also occur in association with rheumatoid arthritis.

Vasculitis

Rheumatoid vasculitis most commonly occurs in those patients with long-standing, seropositive, nodular disease. Varying patterns of vasculitis may be seen depending on the calibre of vessels involved. For example, inflammation of post-capillary venules results in palpable purpura, known as leukocytoclastic vasculitis. Involvement of small arterioles is frequently associated with mild distal sensory neuropathy caused by inflammation of the vasa nervorum. It may also present as small infarcts of the digital pulp, gangrene, skin ulceration, or sclero-malacia perforans. Involvement of medium vessels may result in a condition resembling polyarteritis nodosa, with visceral arteritis and occlusion, which may include coronary, pulmonary, coeliac access, and cerebral vessels. Mononeuritis multiplex may occur and livido reticularis.

Cardiac manifestations

Just as serositis may result in asymptomatic pleural inflammation, similarly pericardial inflammation may be detected by imaging in asymptomatic individuals. It may also present with pain, tamponnade or constriction. Coronary artery disease is a frequently recognised association with rheumatoid arthritis, and a true coronary arteritis may occur, resulting in myocardial infarction. Myocardial disease may result due to diffuse fibrosis or granulomatous lesions, with consequential congestive cardiac failure. Rheumatoid nodules may form in and around the myocardial tissue, resulting in conduction defects or, more rarely, valvular incompetence.

Felty's syndrome

The classic triad of Felty's syndrome is characterised by the occurrence of seropositive rheumatoid arthritis, neutropenia, and splenomegaly. Thrombocytopenia may also occur and severe cases of neutropenia are complicated by recurrent bacterial infections. Felty's syndrome is uncommon, occurring in about 1% of patients, who are not only seropositive but tend to have nodules and other extra-articular manifestations. Nearly all these patients carry the HLA-DR4 gene. Other complications of Felty's syndrome include chronic non-healing ulcers and a greatly increased risk of developing non-Hodgkin's lymphoma. Nodular hyperplasia of the liver has been described, and portal hypertension can result with complicating varices.

Treatment of Felty's syndrome is essentially the same as for patients with active joint disease. In the past, splenectomy was undertaken for those patients suffering severe recurrent bacterial infections. More recently, however, splenectomy has generally been avoided and neutropenia treated if need be with courses of granulocyte-colony-stimulating-factor (G-CSF), with a view to increasing peripheral blood neutrophil counts above 1500 per cubic millimetre. One of the disadvantages of this treatment approach is that it may exacerbate arthritis and vasculitis.

Neurological complications

A number of entrapment neuropathies may occur in the context of rheumatoid arthritis, among the most common being: (i) the median nerve resulting in carpal tunnel syndrome; (ii) the posterior tibial nerve, resulting in tarsal tunnel syndrome; (iii) the ulnar nerve, resulting in cubital tunnel syndrome; and (iv) the posterior interossius branch of the radial nerve.

The troubling neurological sequelae of these neuropathies can usually be treated successfully with decompression surgery. It is, therefore, important to diagnose them correctly and neurophysiological tests can be very helpful for this reason. As well as the relatively rare and sometimes severe sensorimotor mononeuritis multiplex, resulting from vasculitis of the vasa nervorum, a distinct axonal degeneration can occur resulting in a mild symmetrical sensory peripheral neuropathy in a glove and stocking distribution.

Osteoporosis

This complication is seen in a majority of rheumatoid arthritis patients, in particular in the form of juxta-articular osteoporosis thought to be related to local synovitis. Both local and more wide-spread osteoporosis are likely to reflect increased osteoclastic activity under the influence of IL-6 and RANK ligand. Other contributory factors include immobility and use of corticosteroids, although some studies have suggested that reduced disease activity and increased mobility following low-dose prednisolone may actually diminish osteopenia rather than exacerbate it. This remains controversial.

Sjøgren's syndrome

Up to 30% of patients with rheumatoid arthritis develop sicca symptoms typical of secondary Sjøgren's syndrome. However, in distinction to primary Sjøgren's syndrome, although these patients often have a positive anti-nuclear antibody, they generally do not have antibodies to the extractable nuclear antigens Ro and La. Other associated clinical features include marked fatigue and polyarthralgia.

Amyloidosis

Secondary amyloidosis due to the deposition of amyloid AA fibrils has been described in autopsy tissue specimens of up to 10% of patients with rheumatoid arthritis. Deposition may occur in blood vessels, the parenchyma of kidneys, liver, spleen, and gastrointestinal tract. Evidence of amyloidosis may even be found in biopsies taken from the submucosa of the rectum or gingiva. However, symptomatic sequelae of amyloidosis are becoming very uncommon; this may, in part, reflect the trend to much more optimal suppression of the systemic features of rheumatoid arthritis, with combination disease-modifying anti-rheumatic drug (DMARD) therapy, corticosteroids, or even biological therapies. Secondary amyloidosis detected on SAP (serum amyloid P) scanning with radionucleotide-labelled serum amyloid P protein is reported to improve in rheumatoid arthritis patients receiving anti-TNF therapy. In long-standing, poorly controlled rheumatoid arthritis, refractory to therapy, where there is a continuing acute phase response, more serious complications of amyloidosis such as nephrotic syndrome with proteinuria or renal failure may occur.

Laryngeal manifestations

Crico-aretinoid arthritis in varying degrees of severity is relatively common. It may present as pain, dysphagia, or hoarseness, but more rarely in cases of severe disease, as stridor.

Disease expression in seronegative rheumatoid arthritis

The term 'seronegative' implies the absence of detectable rheumatoid factor in patients who, in other respects, fulfil classification criteria for rheumatoid arthritis. It has long been believed that the syndrome of rheumatoid arthritis may represent several different diseases with common phenotypic features. In general, seronegative patients have a better overall prognosis, fewer extra-articular features, and lower mortality. Because the classification criteria are not specific for rheumatoid arthritis, over time it may become clear that some patients labelled as having seronegative rheumatoid arthritis in fact have another form of arthritic condition. It is important to be alert to this possibility as there may be implications for a change in pharmacological management of the condition.

Differential diagnosis

Involvement of the thoracolumbar sacro-iliac or distal interphalangeal joints of the hands is very unusual in rheumatoid arthritis, and often points to an alternative diagnosis such as seronegative spondylo-arthritis, with involvement of sacro-iliac joints, psoriatic arthritis, with involvement of distal interphalangeal joints, or osteoarthritis, with involvement of the lumbar spine and distal interphalangeal joints. Osteoarthritis may present with inflammatory features but, in general, it is distinguished straightforwardly by its distinct joint distribution involving the distal interphalangeal joints of the hand and carpometacarpal joints of the thumb and distinct radiographic features. The comparative features of these two common arthritides are delineated in Table 1.4.

Other differential diagnoses are those of polyarthritis associated with various connective tissue diseases. These include SLE, which may present with a chronic non-deforming polyarthritis. A number of other associated features; for example, photosensitive rash, alopecia, renal or neurological involvement, and Raynaud's phenomenon can usually distinguish it, however. There may also be abnormalities on blood tests to point towards a diagnosis of lupus including haemolytic anaemia, leukopenia, thrombocytopenia, and diagnostic antinuclear antibodies with specificity for double-stranded DNA, Sm, or others. Other connective tissue diseases may also be mistaken for rheumatoid arthritis, including systemic sclerosis, polymyositis, various overlap syndromes, and primary Sjøgren's syndrome. The latter may present with marked fatigue, polyarthralgia or even arthritis, and the presence of rheumatoid factor in high levels. Keratoconjunctivitis sicca is usually present, however, and there may be autoantibodies that help to determine the correct diagnostic label. However, in many cases, in the early phases of disease it will not be possible to categorise the patient with certainty, in which case the term 'undifferentiated early inflammatory arthritis' is helpful.

Polyarthritis may also be the presenting feature of a variety of infectious agents including rubella, parvovirus B-19, Lyme disease, or reactive arthritis associated with infections of the genito-urinary or gastrointestinal tract. In the case of parvovirus B-19 occurring in adults, polyarthritis may be accompanied by transient low-titre rheumatoid factor. However, the arthritis is usually self-limiting. The diagnosis of an infectious arthritis may be confirmed on the basis of detection of IgM antibodies in acute serum samples, with rising IgG antibodies to the inciting agent in convalescent sera. Other differential diagnoses that may cause diagnostic difficulty include polyarticular chronic pyrophosphate arthropathy in more

Table 1.4
Distinction between rheumatoid arthritis and osteoarthritis

	Rheumatoid arthritis	Osteoarthritis
Clinical features		
Osteophytes	Absent	++++
Symmetry	+++	+
Radiographic		
Erosions	+++	Absent
Cysts	++	++
Joint space narrowing	+++	+++
Subchondral sclerosis	+	++++
Osteopenia	+++	Absent

elderly patients. This form of crystal arthritis may be associated with a persistent, but relatively modest, acute phase response and low-titre rheumatoid factor. The distribution of synovitis may be atypical for rheumatoid arthritis and there may also be peri-articular complications. Radiographic appearances in the case of chronic pyrophosphate arthropathy include chondrocalcinosis and the diagnosis can be confirmed when calcium pyrophosphate dihydrate crystals are demonstrated in synovial fluid aspirates. Polyarticular gout is another crystal arthropathy that may be mistaken for rheumatoid arthritis. It is unusual for gout and rheumatoid arthritis to co-exist, although in elderly patients rheumatoid arthritis may co-exist with chronic pyrophosphate disease.

Other differential diagnoses include fibromyalgia, hypermobility syndrome, psoriatic arthritis, haemochromatosis, sarcoidosis, sickle cell disease, primary amyloidosis, and paraneoplastic disease.

Natural history and outcomes

The majority of cases of rheumatoid arthritis present insidiously with joint pain, swelling, and stiffness. The number of involved joints is incremental over weeks to months. About 20% of patients have a subacute onset and 10% present with an acutely severe onset.

It is important to appreciate that the outlook for rheumatoid arthritis has become considerably improved in recent years. A number of factors have contributed to this. For example, as appreciation of the gravity of the social and economic burden imposed by rheumatoid arthritis has grown, so has the recognition that more favourable clinical outcomes are achieved when synovitis is optimally suppressed. In particular, there is now compelling evidence that intervention with disease-modifying combination therapy early in the course of rheumatoid arthritis results in improved remission rates, magnitude of clinical benefit, and slowing of structural damage to joints. In addition, the armamentarium of

potential therapeutics has risen. In the case of untreated disease, or treated rheumatoid arthritis where synovitis is not optimally suppressed, disease activity typically fluctuates over time. This is a feature of the endogenous pathogenic mechanisms of disease but also, in part, a reflection of the variable effectiveness of therapeutic intervention. The major clinical symptoms and signs include joint pain, profound stiffness of the joint, particularly on waking or after immobility, swelling, tenderness to palpation, and restriction of joint movement with loss of functional capability. Many patients also suffer marked fatigue. These features may go through periods of exacerbation lasting weeks or months, with periodic flares in which they become particularly marked. Typically, they will alternate with periods of relative disease quiescence. However, for a subgroup of up to one in five patients with more severe disease expression, the symptoms and signs continue unabated throughout the disease course.

The severity of joint symptoms is very variable. In the majority of cases, there is a direct relationship between the severity of inflammation and structural damage to cartilage, bone, and associated joint structures. This is cumulative over time and largely irreversible even with the most efficacious of current therapies although, as we shall see later, arrest of structural damage to joints can be achieved in a proportion of patients.

Prior to the recent era of more widely available biological therapies, functional deterioration tended to occur rapidly. Long-term outcomes for patients with rheumatoid arthritis have been documented in a number of prospective studies of patients presenting to hospital clinics with recent-onset joint symptoms. Based on data obtained before the early 1990s, it would be expected that about half of patients become moderately disabled within 2 years, and a half would progress to functional class three (limitation in vocational and avocational activities) or functional class four (totally dependent) within 10 years of disease onset (Fig. 1.5).[15] About one-third of patients who

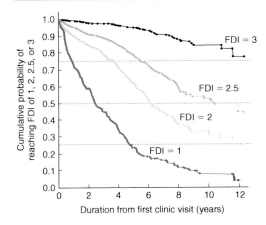

Figure 1.5
The development of disability over time in a group of
rheumatoid arthritis patients studied prior to the early
1990s.
FDI is the functional disease index where 1 = moderate
disability, 2 = more marked disability, 3 = severe
disability and 4 very severe disability.
Reproduced with permission from Wolfe and Cathey.[15]

were in employment at the time of onset of the
condition would have had to leave the
workforce within 5 years. However, patients are
more likely to be able to continue in
employment when their jobs involve less
physical work, where flexible working hours are
possible, and if they have a higher educational
and psychosocial status.

Historical data indicate that the standardised
mortality ratio for rheumatoid arthritis is up to
2.5 times that of age- and sex-matched
individuals without this condition. In the
rheumatoid population as a whole, data
gathered largely prior to the availability of
biological therapies indicated a shortened life
expectation by 5–10 years. The poorest
outcomes are seen in those with most severe
disease. For example, patients with the poorest
functional status and multiple joint
involvement have a 5-year survival rate of 50%
or less. However, optimum suppression of
synovitis with conventional DMARDs or

biological therapy can significantly reduce
disability over time.

Cardiovascular complications account for the
majority (over 40%) of increased mortality in
rheumatoid arthritis. There is also a greatly
increased risk of cancer and lymphoproliferative
malignancies at about 5–8-fold the rate in the
general population. There has been much
debate as to whether this increased risk of
malignancy is associated with the pathogenic
mechanisms responsible for rheumatoid arthritis
itself, or to therapy and, in particular, to the
immunosuppressive effects of drugs such as
methotrexate, cyclosporin, or cyclophosphamide
used in cases of vasculitis and extra-articular
disease. The current consensus is that, in
general, it is the total inflammatory burden
over time that is the major determinate of
increased cancer and lymphoproliferative risk.[16]
Other associations contributing to the increased
mortality in rheumatoid arthritis include renal
disease secondary to amyloidosis,
gastrointestinal haemorrhaging related to non-
steroidal anti-inflammatory drugs (NSAIDs), and
infections, in particular pneumonias. The rate
of infections is increased about 5-fold over that
of the general population. About 10% of deaths
are attributable directly to the rheumatoid
itself. This may be as a result of atlanto-axial
dislocation, extra-articular involvement of the
lungs and heart, primary vasculitis, or therapy
related.

When should primary care practitioners refer patients with inflammatory arthritis to a secondary care specialist?

Rapid referral from primary care to a secondary
care specialist will be indicated when there are
one or more pointers to inflammatory disease.[17]
These include: (i) more than three swollen
joints; (ii) a positive squeeze test (eliciting
marked tenderness on squeezing the
metatarsophalangeal joints or
metacarpophalangeal joints); (iii)
metacarpophalangeal joint or wrist joint
swelling; and (iv) morning joint stiffness
persisting more than 30 minutes.

Not all the above features need necessarily be present to warrant rapid referral; indeed, the heterogeneity of presentation of rheumatoid arthritis is such that it is important to refer any patient in whom an inflammatory polyarthritis is suspected. It is also important to remember that many patients presenting with joint symptoms and signs will either self-medicate with NSAIDs available over the counter, or will be prescribed these drugs by their general practitioner. In many cases, there may be a very good initial response and this does not imply that subsequent referral is unnecessary.

Which tests can usefully be obtained prior to secondary care referral?

The following tests are useful: (i) acute phase markers, *i.e.* erythrocyte sedimentation rate and/or C-reactive protein; (ii) rheumatoid factor; and (iii) radiographs of the hands and feet as erosive change may be seen first at the metatarsophalangeal joints.

Why is early referral so important?

This issue will be discussed in detail in later chapters on the management of rheumatoid arthritis. However, at this point it is useful to note that there is abundant evidence that long-term outcomes are greatly improved when synovitis is optimally suppressed at the earliest stages of disease.[18] Ideally, this would be within 12 weeks of symptom onset. Outcomes are improved both with respect to the symptoms and signs of rheumatoid arthritis, as well as improved outcomes with respect to structural damage to joints. Early intervention also leads to a better chance of sustained remission and preservation of function.

Epidemiology

In numerous epidemiological studies, the prevalence of rheumatoid arthritis is reported as being between 0.8% and 1% of the adult population in cross-sectional studies in western Europe and the US. Female patients outnumber males in a ratio of 3:1. Lower prevalence rates of 0.2– 0.3% have been reported in China and

Japan. In the case of the black population in rural South Africa, the prevalence rate is reported to be about 0.2%, and much lower still in parts of Nigeria. This contrasts with prevalence rates of almost 1% among black populations in urban South Africa and the US. The highest prevalence rates reported in any racial groups are among certain native American Indian tribes, in particular the Pima and Chippewa Indians, with rates exceeding 5%. Estimates of the incidence of rheumatoid arthritis vary considerably, depending on the methodology employed. For example, rheumatoid arthritis incidence estimates in the UK, age-adjusted to the population of England and Wales, are 31 per 100,000 for women and 13 per 100,000 for men, if up to 12 months elapses from symptom onset to application of classification criteria at the baseline assessment by a specialist. However, if up to 5 years elapses from symptom onset to application of the criteria, these estimates rise by 45% for women and 36% for men. In the case of a 5-year lapse between symptom onset and notification to a research registry, followed by cumulative application of classification criteria, estimates rise further still, by 75% for women and 93% for men, reaching figures of 54 per 100,000 for women and 24.5 per 100,000 in men. The highest age-adjusted estimates are probably the most accurate available.[19]

Historical perspective

Garrod first used the term 'rheumatoid arthritis' in his book published in 1859. However, the first clinical description in medical literature is widely attributed to Landre-Bouvais, a physician at the Salpetriere Hospital in Paris in 1800. This too, however, is pre-dated considerably by descriptions of deforming polyarticular disease in classical texts by Galen and others. It is not clear, however, whether these were referring to the syndrome of rheumatoid arthritis as we currently classify it, or other disease such as polyarticular gout.

Archaeological evidence of rheumatoid arthritis in the skeletal remains of native American populations has led to speculation that rheumatoid arthritis spread to Europe following the discovery of the New World.

References

1. Harrison B, Symmons D. Early inflammatory polyarthritis: results from the Norfolk Arthritis Register with a review of the literature. II. Outcome at three years. *Rheumatology* 2000; **39**: 939–49.

2. Machold KP, Stamm TA, Eberl GJ et al. Very recent onset arthritis – clinical, laboratory, and radiological findings during the first year of disease. *J Rheumatol* 2002; **29**: 2278–87.

3. Harrison BJ, Symmons DP, Barrett EM, Silman AJ and the American Rheumatism Association. The performance of the 1987 ARA classification criteria for rheumatoid arthritis in a population based cohort of patients with early inflammatory polyarthritis. *J Rheumatol* 1998; **25**: 2324–30.

4. Saraux A, Berthelot JM, Chales G et al. Ability of the American College of Rheumatology 1987 criteria to predict rheumatoid arthritis in patients with early arthritis and classification of these patients two years later. *Arthritis Rheum* 2001; **44**: 2485–91.

5. Symmons DP, Hazes JM, Silman AJ. Cases of early inflammatory polyarthritis should not be classified as having rheumatoid arthritis. *J Rheumatol* 2003; **30**: 902–4.

6. Visser H, le Cessie S, Vos K, Breedveld FC, Hazes JM. How to diagnose rheumatoid arthritis early: a prediction model for persistent (erosive) arthritis. *Arthritis Rheum* 2002; **46**: 357–65.

7. Arnett FC, Edworthy SM, Bloch DA et al. The American Rheumatism Association 1987 revised criteria for the classification of rheumatoid arthritis. *Arthritis Rheum* 1988; **31**: 315–24.

8. Plant MJ, Jones PW, Saklatvala J, Ollier WE, Dawes PT. Patterns of radiological progression in early rheumatoid arthritis: results of an 8 year prospective study. *J Rheumatol* 1998; **25**: 417–26.

9. Steiner G, Smolen J. Autoantibodies in rheumatoid arthritis and their clinical significance. *Arthritis Res* 2002; **4 (Suppl 2)**: S1–5.

10. Schellekens GA, Visser H, de Jong BA et al. The diagnostic properties of rheumatoid arthritis antibodies recognizing a cyclic citrullinated peptide. *Arthritis Rheum* 2000; **43**: 155–63.

11. Nell VP, Machold KP, Stamm TA et al. Autoantibody profiling as early diagnostic and prognostic tool for rheumatoid arthritis. *Ann Rheum Dis* 2005; **64**:1731–6.

12. Taylor PC. The value of sensitive imaging modalities in rheumatoid arthritis. *Arthritis Res Ther* 2003; **5**: 210–3.

13. Wakefield RJ, Gibbon WW, Conaghan PG et al. The value of sonography in the detection of bone erosions in patients with rheumatoid arthritis: a comparison with conventional radiography. *Arthritis Rheum* 2000; **43**: 2762–70.

14. McQueen FM, Stewart N, Crabbe J et al. Magnetic resonance imaging of the wrist in early rheumatoid arthritis reveals a high prevalence of erosions at four months after symptom onset. *Ann Rheum Dis* 1998; **57**: 350–6.

15. Wolfe F, Cathey MA. The assessment and prediction of functional disability in rheumatoid arthritis. *J Rheumatol* 1991; **18**: 1298–306.

16. Baecklund E, Iliadou A, Askling J et al. Association of chronic inflammation, not its treatment, with increased lymphoma risk in rheumatoid arthritis. *Arthritis Rheum* 2006; **54**: 692–701.

17. Emery P. Treatment of rheumatoid arthritis. *BMJ* 2006; **332**: 152–5.

18. van Aken J, van Dongen H, le Cessie S, Allaart CF, Breedveld FC, Huizinga TW. Comparison of long term outcome of patients with rheumatoid arthritis presenting with undifferentiated arthritis or with rheumatoid arthritis: an observational cohort study. *Ann Rheum Dis* 2006; **65**: 20–5.

19. Wiles N, Symmons DP, Harrison B et al. Estimating the incidence of rheumatoid arthritis: trying to hit a moving target? *Arthritis Rheum* 1999; **42**: 1339–46.

2 Genetics, aetiology and pathogenesis

Genetics
Environmental factors
Synovial pathology and mechanisms of joint destruction
Pathogenesis

Genetics

The initiating cause of rheumatoid arthritis remains unknown. Genetic factors were originally implicated in the aetiopathogenesis of rheumatoid arthritis following the discovery that, in population studies, there is a slight increase in the frequency of rheumatoid arthritis in first-degree relatives of patients, especially if seropositive for rheumatoid factor (Table 2.1) . Familial aggregation studies show the concordance rate for rheumatoid arthritis for monozygotic twins is 30–50%. For dizygotic twins, it is the same as for other sibling pairs at 2–3%. Overall, if one sibling has rheumatoid arthritis, the risk for the unaffected sibling to go on to develop rheumatoid arthritis is about 5–10 times that of someone in the general population. These figures support the concept of a genetic contribution in the pathogenesis of

rheumatoid arthritis, but strongly argue against the proposition that it is the result of a dominant, single-gene disorder. The findings also argue in favour of a relevant environmental trigger.

Genetic analyses indicate that allelic polymorphisms of genes on the short arm of chromosome 6 that code for a hypervariable region of the β-chain of HLA-DR class II molecules are among candidates for involvement in predisposition to rheumatoid arthritis. The discovery first came about with the observation that 60–70% of Caucasian patients with rheumatoid arthritis are HLA-DR positive, compared with 20–25% of control populations. Furthermore, patients with more severe rheumatoid arthritis, especially those with extra-articular complications such as vasculitis and Felty's syndrome, are even more likely to be HLA-DR positive than patients with less aggressive disease confined to the joints.

The immunological significance of HLA class II molecules, expressed on the surface of antigen-presenting cells, lies in their key role in presentation of processed linear peptide antigens of at least nine amino acids to T cells. Antigen is bound to the HLA antigen-binding cleft formed by the α- and β-chains of the HLA class II molecule. This trimolecular HLA antigen complex binds, in turn, to the variable portion of the T-cell receptor. Research studies have defined the sequence of amino acids associated with rheumatoid arthritis as a pentapeptide of amino acid residues from positions 70 to 74, located in the helical wall of the antigen-binding cleft of the HLA-DR β-chain. This sequence, glutamine-arginine or lysine-arginine-alanine-alanine, is known as the 'shared epitope'.[1-3]

The sequence is present on HLA-DR4 subtypes W4 and W14, and on the HLA DR1 subtype DW1, coded by DR B1*0401, *0404, and 0101 genes, respectively. This amino acid sequence is detected in up to 90% of patients of Western European descent with rheumatoid arthritis. The finding is consistent with the hypothesis that these HLA-DR molecules present antigens to T-

Table 2.1
The genetic component of the aetiology of rheumatoid arthritis

General population	~0.8%
Siblings	~3–4%
Non-identical twins	~3–4%
Identical twins	~15%

Conclusion: More than one but less than five genes influence susceptibility and/or disease expression.

cell receptors in a pathogenic process relevant to rheumatoid arthritis. In contrast, negative associations are observed between other HLA-DR4 subtypes and rheumatoid arthritis. These include DW10 and DW13. In DW10 patients, the charged basic amino acids glutamine and arginine in positions 70 and 71 are replaced by the acidic amino acids aspartic and glutamic acid (Table 2.2). In the case of DW13 individuals, arginine is substituted for glutamic acid in position 74. These changes may be sufficient to alter the binding of particular antigens to the HLA cleft. Alternatively, changes in this pentapeptide sequence may influence interactions between the T-cell receptor and the HLA-DR β-chain independently of peptide, in such a way that signals delivered to T cells activate regulatory pathways with protective function rather than arthritogenic pathways.

It may be the case that genes encoding the shared epitope are more useful as markers of disease severity in established rheumatoid arthritis than as markers of disease susceptibility. For example, $DR\beta_1$ *04 genes correlate with seropositive erosive and extra-articular disease. Homozygoticity for $DR\beta_1$ *0401 or $DR\beta_1$ *0404, or when they are combined with each other or with $DR\beta_1$ *0101 (as compound homozygotes), also correlates with more severe disease expression. There is an association between HLA-$DR\beta_1$ alleles carrying the shared epitope and antibodies directed against cyclic citrullinated peptides. Recent data based on studies of populations in North America and The Netherlands suggest that HLA-$DR\beta_1$ alleles encoding the shared epitope do not associate with all patients meeting classification criteria for rheumatoid arthritis; rather, they are specific for those patients with a particular phenotype characterised by production of antibodies to cyclic citrullinated peptide.[4]

Other potential susceptibility genes have been sought away from the HLA-DR locus. Associations with T-cell receptor gene polymorphisms and deletions of immunoglobulin genes have been reported.[5] Other studies have looked for positive or negative correlations between disease severity and gene polymorphisms detected by nucleotide sequencing or microsatellite mapping. These studies have focused on candidate genes coding for proteins known to be involved in the pathogenesis of rheumatoid arthritis, including pro-inflammatory cytokines such as tumour necrosis factor alpha (TNF-α), and anti-inflammatory cytokines such as interleukin 10 (IL-10). These genetic polymorphisms, which may influence the balance of pro- and anti-inflammatory cytokines of relevance for the disease course of rheumatoid arthritis, may be associated with disease severity and also with clinical response to biological therapies targeting TNF-α.[6]

Table 2.2
HLA-DR associations with rheumatoid arthritis defined by $DR\beta_1$ sequence position 70–74

DR type	Sequence					Association
	70	71	72	73	74	
DR4-W4	Q	K	R	A	A	Positive
DR4-W14	Q	R	R	A	A	Positive
DR4-W15	Q	R	R	A	A	Positive
DR1	Q	R	R	A	A	Positive
DR4-W10	D	E	R	A	A	Negative
DR4-W13	Q	K	R	A	E	Negative

Q, glutamine; K, lysine; R, arginine; D, aspartic acid; E, glutamic acid.

Environmental factors

It seems very likely, based on population and twin studies, that non-inherited factors play a role in the aetiology of rheumatoid arthritis as well as a genetic susceptibility component. It is likely that the non-inherited factors will include environmental triggers, and there has been much interest for many years in determining whether the presence of such triggers in a genetically susceptible individual will give rise to immunological abnormalities and, ultimately, to the clinical syndrome of rheumatoid arthritis. Epidemiological studies have addressed these questions by investigating differences in the incidence or prevalence of rheumatoid arthritis in genetically similar populations but in the setting of different environments, for example, urban or rural settings, as well as life-style issues. The findings of these studies are not always easy to interpret, however. For example, in South Africa, there appears to be a higher point prevalence of rheumatoid arthritis in people of the Bantu race living in an urban township area as compared with those in a rural community. However, among Chinese people living in urban Hong Kong, the prevalence of rheumatoid arthritis is low, and certainly not greater than that observed in rural areas. Although the prevalence of rheumatoid arthritis among Bantu people living in urban areas was similar to that expected for a white population in Western countries, the prevalence of rheumatoid arthritis among the black population in Manchester in the UK was actually lower than that of the white population.

Infection

There have also been long-standing interests in the possibility that one or more infections may have a potential role in initiating rheumatoid arthritis. There has been particular interest in a number of viruses including rubella, parvovirus B-19 and Epstein-Barr virus, and in some bacteria including *Proteus* spp., *Mycoplasma* spp., and *Mycobacteria* spp. Human parvovirus B-19 in particular has been proposed as a causative agent for rheumatoid arthritis on the basis of detection of DNA in the synovial tissues of the majority of patients and infrequent finding of DNA in synovial tissues from patients with osteoarthritis and joint trauma. Furthermore, the B-19 antigen BP-1 was found to be specifically expressed in active lesions in synovium of rheumatoid arthritis patients, but not in osteoarthritis or control specimens.[7] However, other, more recent, studies indicate a high frequency of parvovirus B-19 DNA in bone marrow samples from rheumatic patients, indicating a high frequency of persistent infection, but without supporting clinical data to indicate a direct association between this positivity and clinical features of rheumatoid arthritis.[8] Furthermore, the arthritis associated with parvovirus B-19 infection is sporadic and self-limiting, and epidemiological studies do not suggest a classical clustering of new cases anticipated if rheumatoid arthritis were the result of a single infectious agent.

Smoking

There is now compelling evidence that, in a particular genetic context, smoking is a potential trigger for rheumatoid arthritis. Furthermore, when these two factors occur together, they are associated with immunological abnormalities that may considerably antedate the onset of clinical features of rheumatoid arthritis. Using a biobank of about 90,000 archived serum samples from individuals in northern Sweden, it was possible to demonstrate the presence of rheumatoid factor and antibodies to citrullinated peptides up to 10 years before the clinical onset of disease.[9]

Very similar findings have been reported in historical material in a Dutch study, namely that about a quarter of individuals who later developed rheumatoid arthritis had developed antibodies to citrullinated peptides before disease onset, compared with less than 1% of controls. In the Swedish cohort, researchers have asked whether an environmental trigger such as smoking in a genetically susceptible individual might trigger production of antibodies to citrullinated proteins and, subsequently, to features of rheumatoid arthritis. In those patients positive for rheumatoid factor and meeting classification criteria for rheumatoid arthritis, both possession of the shared epitope and smoking are risk factors for seropositive disease, with marked interaction between environmental exposure and the genetic risk factor. Individuals carrying double alleles for the shared epitope, and who are also smokers, are at ~16-fold increased risk of seropositive rheumatoid arthritis, compared with individuals who neither smoke nor carry any copy of the shared epitope genes. In marked contrast, neither of these two risk factors alone nor in combination contributed any risk for the development of seronegative rheumatoid arthritis.[10,11]

Sex hormones

A number of observations point to a role for sex hormones and prolactin in the aetiology of rheumatoid arthritis, including the increased prevalence in females which is most marked before the menopause. Furthermore, the incidence of rheumatoid arthritis increases in the postpartum period and during lactation, whereas the inflammatory component of disease is often markedly improved during pregnancy itself. The oral contraceptive pill is to have a protective effect and postpones the onset of rheumatoid arthritis, presumably because of its progesterone content. In the case of male patients, testosterone levels may be lower than average, and the incidence increases with age as testosterone levels decline. The biological mechanisms behind these observations are not fully understood. They may reflect interplay between cytokine production, sex hormone production, and the hypothalamic–pituitary axis.

Synovial pathology and mechanisms of joint destruction

Infection

Cellular pathology

Rheumatoid joint disease is characterised by synovial hyperplasia with redundant folds, villous projections into the synovial cavity, and tissue oedema.

In healthy joints, the synovial membrane or intima is a fine film, one or two cell layers thick, lining the capsule and having the appearance of 'cling-film' on arthroscopic inspection. The normal intima has no basement membrane and comprises type A and type B synoviocytes without a basement membrane and lying on a bed of loose connective tissue with a network of small blood vessels (the sub-intima). Type A synoviocytes are macrophage-like and type B synoviocytes are of mesenchymal origin and fibroblast-like cells. In the established phase of rheumatoid arthritis, intimal lining hyperplasia becomes prominent, with migration of new type A synoviocytes from the bone marrow into the joint by the bloodstream, and accumulation of type B synoviocytes, either by local proliferation, transmigration of precursor cells from the bone marrow directly into the synovium, or defective cell death. The diseased synovial intimal may be many cell layers deep and coated by a film of fibrin.

Rheumatoid arthritis is characterised by chronic inflammation of synovial joints with synovial proliferation and infiltration by blood-derived cells, in particular, memory T cells, macrophages, and plasma cells, all of which show signs of activation. Luxuriant vasculature is a prominent feature of rheumatoid synovitis, observed as a fine network of vessels over the rheumatoid synovium at arthroscopic inspection of joints.

Angiogenesis is evident on microscopic examination of synovial biopsies from the earliest stages of disease development. Formation of new blood vessels permits a supply of nutrients and oxygen to the augmented inflammatory cell mass, and so contributes to the perpetuation of synovitis. In the chronic phase of disease, capillaries and post-capillary venules are particularly evident in the synovial sublining region. In histological sections, mononuclear and polymorphonuclear leukocytes can sometimes be found in close apposition to vascular endothelium, probably in the process of margination and adhesion prior to migration into the inflamed tissues.

In established disease, the sub-intima is also greatly expanded by newly formed blood vessels and infiltrating mononuclear cells, including T cells, B cells, macrophages, and plasma cells. CD4+ T cells represent the majority at around 50–70%, with macrophages comprising an additional 20%. The cellular infiltrate is often organised into a recognisable architecture comprising perivascular aggregates of CD4 T cells, with a prominent lymphoid follicular structure, some of which may even display germinal centre formation. The interaggregate areas comprise a mixed inflammatory cell population, including dendritic cells, and macrophages expressing HLA class II, CD8+ T cells, activated B cells, and plasma cells.

The cells that accumulate in the sub-intima are recruited to the joints along a chemotactic gradient, including chemotactic cytokines, and also by binding cell adhesion molecules, such as intercellular adhesion molecule 1 (ICAM-1), e-selectin, and VLA 4 on high endothelial venules. By means of a relatively loose binding between e-selectin on activated endothelial cells and its ligand on the surface of intravascular leukocytes, the inflammatory cells are able to roll along the vascular wall until they come to a halt by means of stronger binding to cell adhesion molecules, including VCAM-1 and ICAM-1, prior to diapedesis into the inflamed tissue from the vascular compartment.

Synovial fluid in rheumatoid arthritis

The thickened synovial membrane is bathed in inflammatory synovial fluid, which may be clinically detectable as an effusion. Whereas neutrophils are rarely retained within the subintimal layer, they comprise the majority cell type in synovial fluid. Granulocytes are attracted into the fluid down a gradient of chemotactic factors including leukotriene B_4, platelet activating factor, the C5a fragment of complement, and CXC chemokines such as IL-8 and GRO-α. The total white cell counts are typically between 5000 and 50,000 per cubic millimetre. Rarely, synovial fluid white cell counts can exceed 100,000 cells per cubic millimetre and thus mimic sepsis, which must always be excluded. In addition to neutrophils, CD4+ and CD8+ lymphocytes are present, as well as macrophages, dendritic cells, and synoviocytes. The protein level is elevated and the glucose level may be low, as compared with serum values (40–60% of serum glucose). The fluid is rich in pro-inflammatory cytokines and immune complexes containing rheumatoid factor in the case of seropositive patients. There is local complement consumption, resulting in low haemolytic complement activity, low C3 and C4, with an increase in complement breakdown products.

Pannus

Pannus, which can be defined as synovitis which is adherent to cartilage and locally invasive, is the invasive front of rheumatoid tissue. The destructive lesion typically occurs at the circumferential attachment of the joint capsule, just below and adjacent to the articulate cells at the cartilage–pannus junction, and is comprised of synoviocytes and macrophages, whereas the pannus-invading subchondral bone has abundant osteoclasts. The extracellular matrix damage in this region is caused by several families of enzymes, including serine proteases and cathepsins. Osteoclasts produce cathepsin-K in particular, which is implicated in destruction of bone matrix. Among the most important mediators of tissue destruction are the matrix metalloproteinase enzymes including collagenase, stromelysin, and gelatinase. These can degrade virtually all of the major structural proteins in the joint. Aggrecanase degrades proteoglycan. In addition to cartilage matrix degradation, there is a loss of chondrocyte numbers and reduced chondrocyte activity. Expression of degradative enzymes is regulated by pro-inflammatory cytokines, including IL-1 and TNF-α.

Pathological examination of joint specimens taken at the time of arthroplasty in the later stages of disease has indicated the presence of fibrous tissue replacing regions of destroyed cartilage and bone, suggesting that reparative processes may occur, but without restoration of normal tissue architecture.

Pathogenesis

The initiating cause of rheumatoid arthritis remains unknown. However, over the last two decades there have been significant advances in understanding of pathogenesis, and it is clear that there is inappropriate activation of the immune system resulting in a chronic inflammation and, in most cases, accompanying tissue destruction.

Inflammatory cell recruitment to involved joints

In rheumatoid arthritis, the inflamed synovium is characterised by a mononuclear cell infiltrate and luxuriant vasculature. The increased cell mass is largely accounted for by cells of lymphohaemopoietic origin, indicative of mechanisms allowing inflammatory cell recruitment as well as retention within the

joint. Angiogenesis is key to this process and evident in synovial biopsies from the earliest stages of disease evolution.[12] At arthroscopic inspection of the rheumatoid joint, this increase in vascularity is observed as a fine network of vessels over the rheumatoid synovium. A number of interdependent processes promote angiogenesis in the rheumatoid joint. These include mechanical processes such as the shear stress on the endothelial wall as a result of increased blood flow, as well as a number of pro-angiogenic stimuli released as inflammatory cell products. Many endothelial growth factors are present in the rheumatoid synovium; of these, vascular endothelial growth factor is the most endothelial cell-specific growth factor characterised to date.

Inflammatory cell ingress to the rheumatoid joint is made possible by activation of both limbs of the inflammatory cell recruitment cascade – augmented expression of endothelial cell adhesion molecules permitting binding of lymphocytes, polymorphs, and monocytes, and the action of chemotactic factors which promote the migration of cells into the inflammatory site. These chemotactic factors include representatives of the two families of chemokines, the CXC chemokines such as IL-8 and GRO-α, and CC chemokines such as RANTES (regulated upon activation, T cell-expressed, and secreted), MCP-1 (monocyte chemoattractant protein 1), MIP-1α (macrophage inflammatory protein α), and MIP-1β. Cleaved complement components C3a and

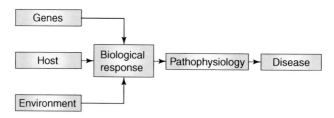

Figure 2.1
The basis of a multigenic syndrome.

C5a present in the rheumatoid joint are also chemotactic for neutrophils, which are retained within joint fluid but generally not within synovial tissue. Some adhesion molecules such as E-selectin are exclusively expressed on the luminal surface of endothelial cells, whereas others including ICAM-1 and VCAM-1 are expressed on activated endothelial cells and other cell types within the inflamed synovium. SDF-1, produced by synovial fibroblasts, is believed to be of importance in T-cell retention and low apoptosis.[13]

Antigen-presenting cells

Presentation of self-antigen to T cells is thought to be central to the pathogenesis of rheumatoid arthritis. A variety of cell types are capable of antigen-presenting cell function. Dendritic cells in particular have attracted much interest in recent years, because of their potent ability to present antigen and, in particular, their unique capacity to activate naive T cells.[14] Dendritic cells are located in anatomical regions where there is a high potential for invasion of pathogens, including the gastrointestinal mucosa and epidermis. In health, dendritic cells play an important role in sampling potential autoantigens and sustaining peripheral tolerance. Dendritic cell populations are also present in rheumatoid synovitis. There is also a predominance of CD4 T cells in proximity to antigen-presenting cells in inflamed rheumatoid synovium.

T cells

T cells are particularly abundant in active rheumatoid arthritis, and may comprise 20–50% of cells in the inflamed synovium. This observation has been interpreted as suggesting an important role for T cells in the pathogenesis of rheumatoid arthritis, and further evidence to support this hypothesis includes the epidemiological association between rheumatoid arthritis and the shared epitope, discussed previously, strongly suggesting a role for (auto) antigen presentation. Furthermore, activated T cells may

regulate osteoclast activation and thus joint destruction.[15] Other lines of evidence supporting the hypothesis that T cells play a role in the pathogenesis of rheumatoid arthritis include the observation that depletion of T cells by thoracic duct drainage or modulation by certain immunosuppressive drugs may give rise to improvement in symptoms and signs of disease. However, despite the association of the MHC class II DRβ_1 susceptibility sequence with rheumatoid arthritis, it is likely that synovial T cells are polyclonal, as significant T-cell receptor oligoclonality has not been demonstrated, and they do not produce IL-2 and interferon-γ (IFN-γ) as would be characteristic of antigen-activated cells. Although there is much evidence for autoimmune processes, no clear-cut initiating autoantigen has been described. Candidate autoantigens that have been investigated include cartilage-derived proteins, peptides derived from HLA class II molecules, citrullinated peptides, and immunoglobulins. Autoimmune responses might also arise as a result of molecular mimicry between epitopes on endogenous molecules and infectious entities if immune tolerance is broken by a process known as 'epitope spreading'. Autoimmunity could also arise when neo-antigens are formed, when molecules released from apoptosing cells become modified by oxidative or enzymatic damage.

Many of the T- and B-cell reactivities to autoantigens in rheumatoid arthritis are not specific for this condition. However, there are notable exceptions, including autoantibodies directed against epitopes on the constant domains of the Fc portion of IgG$_1$ (rheumatoid factor) and citrullinated peptides. It may be that some of these autoreactivities arise as a consequence of the particular pathogenic processes in rheumatoid arthritis and are, therefore, process-specific rather than disease-specific. In fact, post-translational modification of autoantigens such as citrullinated peptides, as well as aberrant antigen processing, may obscure the repertoire of the initiating autoimmune response that might conceivably have preceded clinical disease by many years. It is also possible that any T cells autoreactive against an initiating antigen may in effect be hidden by recruitment and accumulation of other non-specific T cells. T cells in the joint do not proliferate, but increase in number by recruitment and retention.

B cells

The role of lymphocytes in the B-cell lineage is not only important for the generation of immunoglobulins, including rheumatoid factors and other autoantibodies. B cells are also highly efficient antigen-presenting cells that may contribute significantly to T cell responses. This may be by provision of signals needed to activate T cells and rheumatoid factor-producing autoreactive B cells are capable of presenting a variety of antigens to antigen-specific T cells and thereby activating them. B cell-activated T cells, in turn, produce a number of pro-inflammatory cytokines that contribute to disease pathogenesis. In rodent models of rheumatoid arthritis, it may be the case that B cells are more important for the effector phase than for the priming phase of disease initiation.

Activated B cells themselves may also produce cytokines that contribute to joint inflammation and destruction, including TNF-α, IL-6, and lymphotoxin. In particular, B cell-produced lymphotoxin may promote the formation of new tertiary lymphoid structures within the synovium.[16] B-cell cytokines may be produced following antigen binding to a B-cell receptor or binding of the co-stimulatory receptor on B cells by the co-stimulatory ligand on activated T cells, macrophages, or dendritic cells.

Historically, the important role of the B-cell lineage in production of autoantibodies has been well recognised. Rheumatoid factors may be directed to all four IgG subclasses. Blood lymphocytes of rheumatoid patients show selectivity for IgG_1 and IgG_2, while lymphocytes from the synovium tend to produce rheumatoid factors preferentially directed to IgG_3. Rheumatoid factors may form immune

complexes which can be detected within the synovium, together with reduced levels of complement components, implicating these complexes in local disease pathogenesis. Complexes may bind to and activate synovial macrophages which subsequently produce pro-inflammatory cytokines important in disease perpetuation. The clinical efficacy, particularly in seropositive disease, of new biological therapies targeting the B-cell lineage such as Rituximab, which binds the CD20 antigen, emphasise the importance of this cell type in disease pathogenesis, although the mechanism of action of Rituximab is not yet fully understood.

Cytokines

Cytokines are small, short-lived proteins and important mediators of local intercellular communication. They play a key role in integrating responses to a variety of stimuli in immune and inflammatory processes. Cytokines derived from macrophages and fibroblasts are abundant in the rheumatoid synovium. These include IL-1, TNF-α, granulocyte macrophage colony-stimulating factor (GM-CSF), IL-6, and numerous chemo-attractant cytokines known as chemokines. Many of these factors are of importance in regulating inflammatory cell migration and activation. By contrast, given the extent of synovial inflammation and lymphocytic infiltration, factors produced by T cells (e.g. IFN-γ, IL-2, and IL-4) are surprisingly sparsely expressed. However, there are a number of cytokines that cause co-stimulation of T-helper (Th) cells, including IL-7, IL-12, IL-15, and IL-18. The cytokine profile in the synovium of early rheumatoid arthritis presents the classic picture of a Th-1 cell response, as defined by IFN-γ production, and low Th-2 cell activity, as defined by IL-4 production.

Tissue expression of an extensive range of pro-inflammatory cytokines in human synovial samples, regardless of differences in donor disease duration, severity, or even drug therapy, has been confirmed in studies from numerous laboratories. These observations imply that

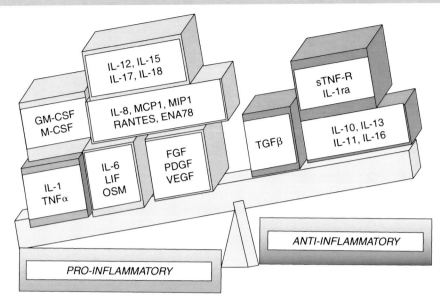

Figure 2.2
The concept of a cytokine disequilibrium. Many cytokines are detectable in rheumatoid synovial tissues, including those with predominantly ant-inflammatory properties. But the net effect is a dominance of pro-inflammatory activity.

there is prolonged expression of cytokines in the rheumatoid joint, contrasting with transient production induced by mitogenic stimuli. This hypothesis was confirmed in the late 1980s, when it was observed that pro-inflammatory cytokines are produced over several days in associated rheumatoid arthritis synovial membrane cell cultures in the absence of extrinsic stimulation. This finding suggested that one or more soluble factors regulating prolonged cytokine synthesis was present within the culture system. The cell cultures comprise a heterogeneous population, producing numerous cytokine and other non-cytokine molecular messengers. Of particular importance, it was observed that the addition of anti-TNF antibodies to the culture strikingly reduced the production of other pro-inflammatory cytokines, including IL-1, GM-CSF, IL-6, and IL-8. Furthermore, using the same rheumatoid arthritis synovial cell culture system, blockade of IL-1 by means of the IL-1 receptor antagonist results in reduced IL-6 and IL-8 production but not that of TNF-α. These

observations led to the concept that TNF-α occupies a dominant position in a pro-inflammatory cytokine hierarchy. TNF-α is a pleiotropic cytokine with biological properties including enhanced synovial proliferation, and production of prostaglandins and metalloproteinases, as well as regulation of other pro-inflammatory cytokines. TNF-α, IL-1, and IL-6 play a role in bone destruction and may also be partly responsible for the peri-articular osteoporosis that is characteristically seen radiographically early in the course of rheumatoid arthritis. TNF-α has been thoroughly validated as a therapeutic target and a number of other cytokine targets are being investigated, with encouraging preliminary data for IL-6 and IL-15.

The predicted clinical success of anti-TNF therapy in rheumatoid arthritis was based on the demonstration of tissue expression of TNF-α in rheumatoid synovial tissue biopsies, *in vitro* experiments employing dissociated synovial cell cultures, and preclinical *in vivo* studies. A number of independent *in vivo* studies demonstrated that antibody therapies blocking bioactivity of TNF-α in murine collagen-induced arthritis, either administered prophylactically or, more importantly, after the onset of disease, were able to ameliorate clinical symptoms and prevent joint destruction. Furthermore, in a murine model over-expressing a human TNF-α transgene modified at its 3'-end to prevent degradation of its messenger RNA, TNF clearly has osteoclastogenic properties associated with a destructive form of polyarthritis developing soon after birth. TNF can stimulate osteoclast formation indirectly by the induction of rank ligand/rank signalling, or directly without induction of rank ligand.[17,18] In the case of the TNF-α transgenic mice, anti-TNF antibodies prevent arthritis and can significantly reverse local bone destruction.[19]

Not only pro-inflammatory cytokines are up-regulated in the rheumatoid synovium, but also multiple anti-inflammatory mediators, although at a level insufficient to suppress the inflammatory component of disease completely. Examples include the abundant expression of IL-10, IL-13, and TGF-β both in latent and active form. Naturally occurring cytokine inhibitors such as IL-1 receptor antagonist (IL-1ra) and soluble TNF receptors (the specific inhibitors of IL-1 and TNF-α, respectively) are also up-regulated in the rheumatoid joint. These observations gave rise to the concept of a cytokine disequilibrium existing in the chronic inflammatory situation in rheumatoid synovium. It may, in part, account for the relapsing and remitting nature of the disease presentation.

Advances in the understanding of the role of cytokines in the immunopathogenesis of rheumatoid arthritis have led to two potential approaches to cytokine modulation as a means of therapeutic intervention: first, inhibition of dominant pro-inflammatory cytokines such as TNF-α or IL-6; or second, augmentation of the inadequate anti-inflammatory activity of certain cytokines or naturally occurring cytokine inhibitors, for example, soluble TNF receptors or IL-1ra. It is now established that the long-term use of several biological agents targeting TNF-α give rise to sustained improvements in symptoms and signs of rheumatoid arthritis. This will be discussed in detail in Chapter 8.

References

1. Gregersen PK, Silver J, Winchester RJ. The shared epitope hypothesis. An approach to understanding the molecular genetics of susceptibility to rheumatoid arthritis. *Arthritis Rheum* 1987; **30**: 1205–13.

2. Winchester RJ, Gregersen PK. The molecular basis of susceptibility to rheumatoid arthritis: the conformational equivalence hypothesis. *Springer Semin Immunopathol* 1988; **10**: 119–39.

3. Hammer J, Gallazzi F, Bono E *et al*. Peptide binding specificity of HLA-DR4 molecules: correlation with rheumatoid arthritis association. *J Exp Med* 1995; **181**: 1847–55.

4. Huizinga TW, Amos CI, van der Helm-van Mil AH *et al*. Refining the complex rheumatoid arthritis phenotype based on specificity of the HLA-DRB1 shared epitope for antibodies to citrullinated proteins. *Arthritis Rheum* 2005; **52**: 3433–8.

5. Olee T, Yang PM, Siminovitch KA *et al*. Molecular basis of an autoantibody-associated restriction fragment length polymorphism that confers susceptibility to autoimmune diseases. *J Clin Invest* 1991; **88**: 193–203.

6. Padyukov L, Lampa J, Heimburger M *et al*. Genetic markers for the efficacy of tumour necrosis factor blocking therapy in rheumatoid arthritis. *Ann Rheum Dis* 2003; **62**: 526–9.

7. Takahashi Y, Murai C, Shibata S *et al*. Human parvovirus B19 as a causative agent for rheumatoid arthritis. *Proc Natl Acad Sci USA* 1998; **95**: 8227–32.

8. Lundqvist A, Isa A, Tolfvenstam T, Kvist G, Broliden K. High frequency of parvovirus B19 DNA in bone marrow samples from rheumatic patients. *J Clin Virol* 2005; **33**: 71–4.

9. Rantapaa-Dahlqvist S, de Jong BA, Berglin E *et al*. Antibodies against cyclic citrullinated peptide and IgA rheumatoid factor predict the development of rheumatoid arthritis. *Arthritis Rheum* 2003; **48**: 2741–9.

10. Padyukov L, Silva C, Stolt P, Alfredsson L, Klareskog L. A gene-environment interaction between smoking and shared epitope genes in HLA-DR provides a high risk of seropositive rheumatoid arthritis. *Arthritis Rheum* 2004; **50**: 3085–92.

11. Klareskog L, Stolt P, Lundberg K *et al*. A new model for an etiology of rheumatoid arthritis: smoking may trigger HLA-DR (shared epitope)-restricted immune reactions to autoantigens modified by citrullination. *Arthritis Rheum* 2006; **54**: 38–46.

12. Taylor PC. Serum vascular markers and vascular imaging in assessment of rheumatoid arthritis disease activity and response to therapy. *Rheumatology (Oxford)* 2005; **44**: 721–8.

13. Buckley CD, Amft N, Bradfield PF *et al*. Persistent induction of the chemokine receptor CXCR4 by TGF-beta 1 on synovial T cells contributes to their accumulation within the rheumatoid synovium. *J Immunol* 2000; **165**: 3423–9.

14. Banchereau J, Steinman RM. Dendritic cells and the control of immunity. *Nature* 1998; **392**: 245–52.

15. Kong YY, Feige U, Sarosi I *et al*. Activated T cells regulate bone loss and joint destruction in adjuvant arthritis through osteoprotegerin ligand. *Nature* 1999; **402**: 304–9.

16. Lund FE, Garvy BA, Randall TD, Harris DP. Regulatory roles for cytokine-producing B cells in infection and autoimmune disease. *Curr Dir Autoimmun* 2005; **8**: 25–54.

17. Azuma Y, Kaji K, Katogi R, Takeshita S, Kudo A. Tumor necrosis factor-alpha induces differentiation of and bone resorption by osteoclasts. *J Biol Chem* 2000; **275**: 4858–64.

18. Kobayashi K, Takahashi N, Jimi E *et al*. Tumor necrosis factor alpha stimulates osteoclast differentiation by a mechanism independent of the ODF/RANKL-RANK interaction. *J Exp Med* 2000; **191**: 275–86.

19. Taylor PC, Feldmann M. Rheumatoid arthritis. In: Ganten D, Ruckpaul K. (eds) *Encyclopaedic Reference of Genomics and Proteomics in Molecular Medicine*. Berlin: Springer, 2006; ISBN: 3-540-44244-8.

20. Smith JB, Haynes MK. Rheumatoid arthritis – a molecular understanding. *Ann Intern Med*. 2002; **136**: 908–22.

3 Assessment of disease activity and response to therapy

Introduction
Assessment of symptoms and signs of
    arthritis
Assessment of structural damage
Assessment of function
Prognostic factors
Criteria for referral of new patients
    following presentation in primary
    care
Summary

Introduction

As discussed in Chapter 1, the presentation and clinical course of rheumatoid arthritis is highly variable between individuals. Furthermore, for any given individual the disease course may also vary in its intensity over time. The symptoms and signs of rheumatoid arthritis cover a wide spectrum, varying from pain, stiffness, swelling, and functional impairment, to more constitutional complaints such as general malaise and profound fatigue. With the passage of time there may be progressive joint destruction and accompanying functional loss. As a result of this variety in disease expression, a large number of outcome variables have been used in recent decades in order to evaluate disease activity, presence of remission, response to therapy, progression of structural damage to joints, and functional status. In part, these evaluations have evolved in order to allow a robust and meaningful interpretation of the therapeutic benefit of new treatment interventions in the context of clinical trials. However, in recent years, it has become increasingly evident that reliable assessment of

disease activity is an important tool in optimising the management of patients with rheumatoid arthritis and ensuring the most favourable outcomes.

Assessment of symptoms and signs of arthritis

Symptoms are assessed by taking a descriptive history and also by attempting to quantify their severity. Similarly, signs of rheumatoid arthritis are documented following a careful examination. Synovial thickening is detected on palpation as a spongy or boggy feel, and tenderness is elicited by squeezing an affected joint. It is always best to do this gently in the first instance! Other classical signs of inflammation such as erythema or raised temperature overlying the affected joint are not as prominent or readily quantifiable on clinical examination alone. Joint effusions can be demonstrated by fluctuation. As the condition progresses, deformities may advance and subluxed surfaces of bones may falsely give the impression of bony swelling. This is particularly evident at the heads of the metacarpals in the hands, the ulnar styloid, and the distal radius at the wrist. There have been a number of approaches to quantifying the severity of these features and some of the most widely used will be discussed below.

The ACR core data set and response criteria

Up until the early 1990s, clinical trials in rheumatoid arthritis were characterised by the use of many different outcome measures, ranging from evaluation of the number of involved joints to grip-strength measurements and laboratory measures. The need for better standardisation led to development of the American College of Rheumatology (ACR) core data set of measures for rheumatoid arthritis clinical trials.[1]

The ACR core data set includes seven measures: three of these are by an assessor – swollen joint count, tender joint count, and physician assessment of global status; three are by patient self-report – physical function, pain, and global status; and one acute phase reactant – either ESR or CRP. In addition to these seven measures, radiographs of the hands and feet are included if a clinical study is of 1 year duration or longer.

ACR preliminary definition of improvement

Further analyses led to the ACR preliminary definition of improvement[2] as follows:

> At least 20% in both the tender and swollen joint counts, as well as three of the five additional core set measures

This definition subsequently became known as the ACR20 response. Higher thresholds for improvement, such as ACR50 and ACR70,[3] have also been described and increasingly used in recent years with the advent of biological therapies demonstrating high levels of efficacy.

The ACR core data set and the 20%, 50%, and 70% improvement criteria have been thoroughly validated and widely used in the context of clinical studies. They allow recognition of significant differences in the efficacy of test versus comparator treatments in clinical trials of new agents for rheumatoid arthritis, and have undoubtedly helped rheumatologists and regulatory agencies to interpret the findings of clinical studies more meaningfully.

The ACR N index

Unlike the ACR 20%, 50%, and 70% response criteria, the ACR N index is a continuous variable derived from the ACR core data set. It is a more sensitive tool for distinguishing therapeutic benefit from an active comparator compound in the context of clinical trials. Differences between baseline and the end-point are calculated for each of the seven measures in the core set. The ACR N is defined as the minimum figure based on the percentage change in swollen joints, tender joints, and the median of the other five core data set measures. An example is given in Figure 3.1. It is thus a conservative measure of improvement. As a continuous index, the ACR N can also be used to indicate deterioration in disease status, which is not possible using the ACR improvement criteria.

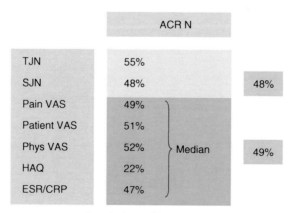

Conclusion: ACR N = 48%

Figure 3.1
Calculation of ACR N.

The disease activity score and the EULAR response criteria

In contrast to the ACR improvement criteria, the EULAR (European League Against Rheumatism) response criteria are based on the disease activity score (DAS), an index using only three or four core set variables. The EULAR and ACR response criteria also differ in a number of other respects. In particular, the EULAR response criteria were developed to distinguish between high and low disease activity, as opposed to demonstrating differences between active and comparator or placebo treatment; the EULAR response criteria define improvement on the basis of significant change and the level of disease activity reached, as opposed to relative change; and the EULAR criteria define three categories of improvement.

Disease activity score

The disease activity score is derived from a formula based on information concerning the number of swollen joints, the number of tender joints, the acute phase response with or without the patient's own assessment of global health status based on a 100-mm visual analogue scale. Various formulae have been derived, depending on the numbers of joints assessed and whether ESR or CRP is used as the acute phase reactant. This composite score gives rise to a continuous measure of rheumatoid inflammation.

The original version of the DAS (DAS44) was developed based on a swollen joint count evaluating 44 joints and the Ritchie index, a graded tender joint count frequently used in Europe. The formulae for calculation of the original disease activity score, based on either three or four variables, is given below:

> DAS44 score with four variables = 0.53938 × square root of Ritchie articular index + 0.06465 × number of swollen joints out of 44 assessed, plus 0.33 multiplied by the Napierian logarithm of the ESR + 0.00722 × the patient assessment of general health on a 100-mm visual analogue scale

> The DAS44 score based on three variables = 0.53938 × the square root of the Ritchie articular index + 0.06465 × the number of swollen joints out of 44 assessed plus 0.33 multiplied by the Napierian logarithm of the ESR + 0.224

The DAS28 is also a composite score based on three or four variables, but in this case the swollen joint count is based on a set of 28 joints assessed. The same joint set is assessed for tenderness in an all-or-nothing manner, without any gradation. The DAS28 score ranges from 0 to 10 and is widely used in clinical practice as well as clinical trials.

> Formulae for calculation of the DAS28 with four variables: 0.56 × square root of the tender joint count out of 28 assessed + 0.28 × square root of the swollen joint count out of 28 assessed, + 0.7 × the Napierian logarithm of the ESR + 0.014 × patient assessment of global health on a 100 mm visual analogue scale
> $$0.56*\sqrt{(t28)} + 0.28*\sqrt{(sw28)} + 0.70*Ln(ESR) + 0.014*GH$$

> Formulae for calculation of the DAS28 based on three variables is calculated as follows: 0.56 × the square root of the tender joint count out of 28 assessed, plus 0.28 × the square root of the swollen joint count of 28 assessed, plus 0.7 × the Napierian logarithm of the ESR; then that entire formula is multiplied by 1.08, and to that is added 0.16
> $$[0.56*\sqrt{(t28)} + 0.28*\sqrt{(sw28)} + 0.70*Ln(ESR)]*1.08 + 0.16$$

There is a high correlation between the modified DAS28 disease activity score with the original DAS at 0.97, and the DAS28 has the same capacity to differentiate between high and low disease activity patients.[4]

The EULAR response criteria use the individual change in DAS and the level of DAS reached to classify clinical trial participants or patients receiving a new therapy as good, moderate, or non-responders depending on the lowest DAS

Table 3.1
The EULAR response criteria using the DAS28

Lowest DAS achieved		DAS28 improvement	
	> 1.2	> 0.6 and ≤ 1.2	≤ 0.6
DAS28 ≤ 3.2	Good response		
3.2 < DAS28 ≤ 5.1		Moderate response	
DAS28 > 5.1			No response

DAS improvement is defined as baseline DAS minus DAS at the point of evaluation.

score achieved and the change in DAS between baseline and the point of evaluation[5] as indicated in Table 3.1.

The performance of the EULAR response criteria has been validated in clinical trials, and compares similarly with ACR improvement criteria. It has often been the case that one set of criteria is used as a primary end-point and the other as a secondary end-point. The EULAR response criteria include not only change in disease activity, but also current disease activity. Thus a change of 1.2 in the DAS28 score is considered significant and represents twice the measurement error. However, in order to be classified as a good responder, a patient must also reach a low disease activity with a DAS28 of less than 3.2.

Use of the DAS 28 in clinical practice

In recent years, much evidence has emerged to indicate that rheumatoid inflammation should be controlled as early as possible, as completely as possible, and that control should be maintained over the long term while taking care to observe appropriate safety precautions. In practice,[6] in order to achieve optimal control of rheumatoid inflammation or even sustained remission with respect to the pharmacological intervention employed, it is essential to review patients regularly and undertake a systematic and quantitative evaluation of disease activity. The DAS28 is now widely used for this purpose and is calculated automatically when the three or four variables involved are entered into a computer in the clinic. A score of greater than 5.1 represents a high level of disease activity;

a score of less than 5.1 and greater than 3.2, moderate disease activity; a score of 3.2 to 2.6, near remission; and a score of less than 2.6 represents remission.

> **Learning point**
> Interpretation of DAS 28 scores
>
> DAS28 > 5.1 represents a high level of disease activity
>
> DAS28 < 5.1 and > 3.2 represents a moderate disease activity
>
> DAS28 < 3.2 and > 2.6 represents near remission
>
> DAS28 < 2.6 represents remission

It is important to emphasise that the DAS28 can be used to support clinical decision making with regard to therapy, but that it does not substitute for a careful history and examination, taking into account the global needs of the patient. For example, the DAS28 is widely used to monitor response to biological therapies and, in some instances, dose titration. Superior outcomes have been demonstrated in clinical studies of combination disease-modifying anti-rheumatic drug (DMARD) therapy, where treatment strategy is based on drug escalation according to a protocol designed to maintain a low DAS score.[7] This issue will be discussed further in the chapters on therapy.

Remission criteria

Remission criteria define the absence of disease activity or at least a very low level of disease activity. Given that the natural history of the inflammatory burden is to fluctuate in rheumatoid arthritis, to be clinically meaningful, remission criteria need to be followed over time to see if they are maintained.

The published American Rheumatism Association (ARA) remission criteria comprise six assessments, all of which should be within the normal range for more than 2 months. These six criteria are: joint pain by history, joint tenderness, joint or tendon sheath swelling, ESR, fatigue, and early morning stiffness (which should be absent or not exceeding 15 minutes). It will be noted that two of the six variables are not included in the validated core set, and that the final outcome is dichotomous. As a consequence, a small change in overall disease activity may have a disproportionately large impact on the allocated class for the patient. These represent very strict criteria that are rarely used in clinical practice, in part because of the inclusion of fatigue. When considering the definition of remission, some clinical investigators have suggested that an ACR70 response approximates to remission, in particular if this magnitude of response is maintained over time. However, in general, an ACR 70% response does not represent true remission, although it may approximate to a near remission.

Remission has also been defined on the basis of a continuous variable of disease activity such as the disease activity score and, in particular, the cumulative disease activity over a given time period. In a prospective follow-up study of patients with early onset rheumatoid arthritis, a comparison was made between the ARA remission criteria and the disease activity score. For the original DAS, a score of less than 1.6 corresponded with remission, as defined by the ARA criteria, and for the DAS28, a score of less than 2.6. However, it should be noted that the original DAS is a more conservative measure of remission than the DAS28 because of differences in the group of joints assessed for swelling and tenderness. Although the DAS and DAS28 remission criteria perform well on a group level, they do not absolutely define remission on an individual patient basis, although the score represents a very useful pointer to the overall level of disease activity.[8]

Assessment of structural damage

Persistent disease activity in rheumatoid arthritis is often accompanied by progression of structural damage to joints, although the rate and extent of damage is highly variable. Evaluation of disease activity and structural damage to joints in rheumatoid arthritis is essential in both routine clinical management and clinical trials. Imaging technologies are required to assess and quantify structural damage to joints. Conventional radiography is the most widely used imaging modality and has standardised methods for interpretation. There are also limitations, including the use of ionising radiation and projectional superimposition that can obscure erosions and mimic cartilage loss, as an inevitable consequence of representing a three-dimensional structure in only two planes.

Quantification of structural damage in the context of clinical trials requires experienced readers and the methods can be time-consuming. Change in radiographs cannot be reliably determined in less than 6–12 months. Newer imaging modalities including MRI and ultrasonographic techniques emphasise the inadequacy of conventional radiography for soft tissue assessment in rheumatoid arthritis. Recent research has focused on standardising these newer imaging technologies and it is likely that they will be increasingly used as sensitive clinical tools with the potential to detect early changes in inflammatory processes and joint destruction that may ultimately reduce clinical trial size and duration.[9]

Radiographic assessment

In many clinical trials, radiographic progression is assessed by reference to standardised images of the hands and feet. Many studies employ the

Sharp or modified Sharp scoring system, in which erosions and joint space narrowing are scored separately. Other researchers have questioned the necessity of scoring both these components, however, and the Larsen index, which has also been widely used, places much less emphasis on joint space narrowing.

The Larsen method scores radiological appearances of joints in the hands, wrists, and feet, compared to a set of reference films for each joint. The joints scored on each side are the first IP joints, the second to fifth PIP joints, and the first to fifth MCP joints in the hand; the first interphalangeal joints and second to fifth MCP joints in the feet; and the wrist as one joint. The range of scores for each joint is 0–5: 0, normal appearance; 1, slight abnormality; 2, definite early abnormality; 3, medium destructive abnormality; 4, severe destructive abnormality; and 5, mutilating abnormality. In calculating the total Larsen's score, all individual joint scores are summed after multiplying the wrist scores by 5. The maximum total score, or Larsen index, is 200 per patient.[10]

The Sharp score, or modified versions of the Sharp score such as the van der Heijde modification, are increasingly used because of its greater sensitivity to change. In the Sharp system, the small joints in the hands and feet were selected for scoring because these are involved in more than 90% of rheumatoid arthritis patients. In the composite scoring method of Sharp and its modifications, erosions and joint space narrowing are scored separately. In the Sharp method, 17 joints are scored in each hand and wrist and six in the feet for erosions; in the van der Heijde modification, 16 joints are scored in the hands and wrists and six in the feet. By the Sharp method, erosions are scored on a 0–5 scale. When erosions are distinct, they are scored as the number of erosions per joint. A score of 5 represents extensive destruction of a joint. When erosions are not distinct, the number of quadrants that contain erosions are counted and scored one point each. If the erosion is confluent, the extent of the involvement is estimated and one

point is assigned for each quintile involved. The Sharp method scores both hands and feet by the same scale.[11] The van der Heijde modification scores hands on the same scale but joints of the feet on a scale of 0–10. The range of scores for erosions is 0–170 or 0–160 for the hands by the Sharp and van der Heijde modification methods, respectively. For the feet, the range is 0–60 by the Sharp scale and 0–120 by the van der Heijde modification scale.[12]

Joint space narrowing is scored on a scale of 0–4. A normal joint with no narrowing is assigned a score of 0; asymmetrical or minimal narrowing is scored as 1; narrowing of 25–60% is scored as 2; narrowing of 60–99% is scored as 3, and a score of 4 represents no visible joint space and presumed ankylosis. The range of joint space narrowing scores for 16 joints in hands and wrists used in the Sharp method is 128 and for five joints in each foot is 40. The van der Heijde method uses the same scale of 0–4 to score 15 joints in each hand and wrist and five in each foot. Thus the range of total scores, the sum of erosion and joint space narrowing, is 398 for the Sharp method and 440 for the van der Heijde modification.

Assessment of function

Evaluation of patient function and disability by means of patient self-reported assessment (rather than physician assessment) has become standard in the context of randomised clinical trials as well as in clinical research. The most commonly used assessment tool for functional disability is the Stanford Health Assessment Questionnaire (HAQ) and its derivatives.[13] The HAQ and similar questionnaires primarily measure function and health-related quality of life. However, it should be noted that such questionnaires do not discriminate between the extent of functional impairment due to currently active disease (that is process-related and, therefore, potentially reversible) and the inevitable sequelae of long-term irreversible joint destruction.

The original HAQ comprises a series of 20 questions in eight different categories. Each question is assigned a score as follows: 0, no difficulty; 1, some difficulty; 2, much difficulty or need for assistance; 3, unable to perform.

The highest score in each category represents the final score for that particular category and the average of the scores for all eight categories yields the total HAQ score on a scale of 0–3. An improvement of 0.25 or more in HAQ score is considered to be clinically meaningful. The HAQ, therefore, reflects both disease process and outcome, and has been well validated as a clinical tool.[14] However, the HAQ score has its limitations as a tool for assessment of patient function. For example, the overall score does not indicate which particular area of health or daily activities constitutes a priority for improvement for any given individual. Furthermore, health preferences and perception of change in status may differ between patients and physicians. Thus, it is possible to see an overall improvement in HAQ score that is not necessarily accompanied by a subjective improvement in the health domain of greatest importance to the patient.

In general, HAQ scores indicate worsening function with increasing disease duration. It is important to remember, however, that several factors impact on functional capability. These include disease activity, cumulative structural

damage to joints, and psychosocial issues (Fig. 3.2).[15,26] In the early stages of disease, in particular, there is a high correlation between disability and inflammation and little clear-cut relationship to radiographic damage (Fig. 3.3).[16] However, as the disease becomes more established and time passes, structural damage becomes a major determinant of functional disability. These observations reflect the fact that the increases in radiographic scores over the short-term, although significant, are insufficient to impact on function. Moreover, standard radiographic assessments are of the hands and feet, although in many cases large-joint damage accounts for a more substantial proportion of disability reflected in the HAQ score.

Prognostic factors

Early identification of patients with rheumatoid arthritis and, in particular, those likely to assume a more rapidly destructive form of disease is important because of the possible benefit from early aggressive intervention with disease-modifying agents or biological therapies. This realisation has prompted the investigation and measurement of numerous biological markers, which may be molecules measured in blood or joint fluid, genetic markers, or imaging markers that may serve as

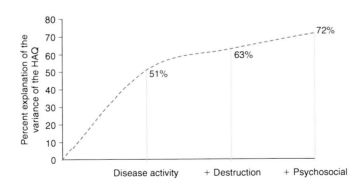

Figure 3.2
Disability as a function of disease activity, destruction, and psychosocial function. From Drossaers-Bakker et al.[26] reprinted with permission of Wiley-Liss, Inc., a subsidiary of John Wiley & Sons, Inc. (© 1999 John Wiley & Sons, Inc.)

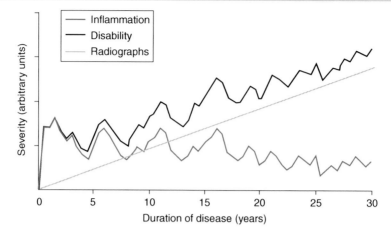

Figure 3.3
There is a high correlation between disability and inflammation in early rheumatoid arthritis. Reproduced from Kirwan[16] with permission.

indicators of prognosis and response to therapy. Many potential markers such as those listed in Table 3.2 reproducibly give prognostic information on a cohort level. However, few of the currently available markers are sufficiently accurate to inform appropriate management decisions on an individual-patient basis. For this reason, there is much active research interest in defining more accurate prognostic markers that could be more easily employed in a routine clinical setting.

Many studies have noted an association between the presence of the HLA-DRβ_1 shared epitope and the severity of radiographic bone damage in rheumatoid arthritis, although this association has not been observed in all cohorts studied. Some investigators report that there is no apparent association between the presence of the shared epitope and radiographic damage in seropositive patients with long-standing rheumatoid arthritis, but there is such an association in seronegative patients, although radiographic outcome is generally less severe.[17] The findings of cohort studies may also be confounded by the effect of treatment on radiographic progression.

Rheumatoid factor is a well-established prognostic test and many studies have confirmed that it is a major predictor of

radiographic bone damage.[18,19] In a study from the UK based on the Norfolk Arthritis Registry, patients with a rheumatoid factor titre greater than 1 in 160 by latex were 2.3 times more likely to have worsening of their Larsen's scores over 5 years than those who were seronegative.[20] Similarly, several studies have demonstrated that antibodies to cyclic citrullinated peptides are of prognostic value for radiographic progression. In a recent study of an early rheumatoid arthritis cohort from The Netherlands, the presence of anti-CCP antibodies at baseline was predictive of radiographic progression after 2 years, with an odds ratio of 14.8.[21]

Although several laboratory measures have been shown to predict a more severe disease course in cohort studies, their positive predictive value is generally not strong enough to inform therapeutic decisions reliably on an individual basis in daily clinical practice. Serial measures of the DAS28 are particularly strong predictors of physical disability and radiographic progression, with an accuracy that increases with cumulative scores over longer sampling intervals.

The presence of radiographic erosions at presentation is predictive of subsequent joint damage. In the early phase of rheumatoid arthritis, ultrasonography is about 6 times more

Table 3.2
Factors predictive of a less favourable outcome in rheumatoid arthritis

Socio-economic and demographic factors	low socio-economic status, fewer years of formal education, female sex, older age
Immunogenetic factors	HLA, $DR\beta_1$ susceptibility sequence
Disease-related factors	insidious disease onset, large number of involved joints, early development of erosions, functional disability, presence of extra-articular features
Clinical laboratory factors	elevated ESR or CRP, seropositivity for rheumatoid factor, thrombocytosis, elevated IL-6

sensitive than conventional radiography for detection of erosions in the small joints of the hand.[22] In future clinical studies it may be possible to stratify patients according to the degree of baseline joint damage as assessed by grey-scale ultrasound.

Many other genetic, serological, and imaging biomarkers are in the stage of experimental evaluation and are not yet widely available. These include serum markers of cartilage turnover, such as cartilage oligomeric matrix protein (COMP),[23] polymorphisms of macrophage migration inhibitory factor,[24] and quantitative vascular imaging of hand joints by power Doppler ultrasonography.[25] In the future, for prognostic tests to have clinical utility, they must be readily available, and based on simple sampling such as a blood test or non-invasive imaging. In a condition with such a heterogeneous clinical expression, it is unlikely that a single variable will have a useful predictive role on an individual patient basis in daily clinical practice, and it is more likely that a panel of markers will be necessary.

Criteria for referral of new patients following presentation in primary care

A rapid referral to a specialist rheumatologist is strongly recommended if a primary care practitioner sees a patient where any of the following features are present: (i) three or more swollen joints; (ii) swelling involving the hand joints; or (iii) joint stiffness in the morning that lasts for 30 minutes or longer.

Ideally, rheumatologists would like to see patients with inflammatory arthritis within the first 12 weeks of symptom onset. Where appropriate, treatment with a disease-modifying, anti-rheumatic drug can be initiated early and this can dramatically improve the long-term prospects for patients.

The clinical presentation of rheumatoid arthritis is exceedingly variable; therefore, correct diagnosis in the early stages can be very difficult. Early referral is strongly recommended for any patient in whom rheumatoid arthritis is suspected. Suggested criteria on which to base a referral decision are discussed in Chapter 2. It should also be emphasised that many patients will respond well to early introduction of NSAIDs and a significant symptomatic improvement is not a reason to delay referral. As discussed in following chapters, NSAIDs may improve symptoms and signs but have no effect on tissue destruction, hence the importance of early referral for consideration of therapeutic intervention known to retard or even prevent joint damage.

Summary

Assessment of symptoms and signs, the presence of remission, structural damage and function are all important for clinical trials in order to evaluate the benefits of new therapies in each of these domains. Similarly, assessment of these parameters has a place in routine clinical practice in order to guide pharmacological management decisions with a view to optimising outcomes.

References

1. Felson DT, Anderson JJ, Boers M et al. and the Committee on Outcome Measures in Rheumatoid Arthritis Clinical Trials. The American College of Rheumatology preliminary core set of disease activity measures for rheumatoid arthritis clinical trials. Arthritis Rheum 1993; 36: 729–40.

2. Felson DT, Anderson JJ, Boers M et al. and the American College of Rheumatology. Preliminary definition of improvement in rheumatoid arthritis. Arthritis Rheum 1995; 38: 727–35.

3. Felson DT, Anderson JJ, Lange ML, Wells G, LaValley MP. Should improvement in rheumatoid arthritis clinical trials be defined as fifty percent or seventy percent improvement in core set measures, rather than twenty percent? Arthritis Rheum 1998; 41: 1564–70.

4. Fransen J, van Riel PL. The Disease Activity Score and the EULAR response criteria. Clin Exp Rheumatol 2005; 23 (Suppl 39): S93–9.

5. van Gestel AM, Prevoo ML, van't Hof MA, van Rijswijk MH, van de Putte LB, van Riel PL. Development and validation of the European League Against Rheumatism response criteria for rheumatoid arthritis. Comparison with the preliminary American College of Rheumatology and the World Health Organization/International League Against Rheumatism Criteria. Arthritis Rheum 1996; 39: 34–40.

6. Wolfe F, Cush JJ, O'Dell JR et al. Consensus recommendations for the assessment and treatment of rheumatoid arthritis. J Rheumatol 2001; 28: 1423–30.

7. Grigor C, Capell H, Stirling A et al. Effect of a treatment strategy of tight control for rheumatoid arthritis (the TICORA study): a single-blind randomised controlled trial. Lancet 2004; 364: 263–9.

8. Prevoo ML, van Gestel AM, van't Hof MA, van Rijswijk MH, van de Putte LB, van Riel PL. Remission in a prospective study of patients with rheumatoid arthritis. American Rheumatism Association preliminary remission criteria in relation to the disease activity score. Br J Rheumatol 1996; 35: 1101–5.

9. Taylor PC. The value of sensitive imaging modalities in rheumatoid arthritis. Arthritis Res Ther 2003; 5: 210–3.

10. Larsen A, Dale K, Eek M. Radiographic evaluation of rheumatoid arthritis and related conditions by standard reference films. Acta Radiol Diagn (Stockh) 1977; 18: 481–91.

11. Sharp JT. An overview of radiographic analysis of joint damage in rheumatoid arthritis and its use in meta-analysis. J Rheumatol 2000;27: 254–60.

12. van der Heijde D. How to read radiographs according to the Sharp/van der Heijde method. J Rheumatol 2000; 27: 261–3.

13. Fries JF, Spitz P, Kraines RG, Holman HR. Measurement of patient outcome in arthritis. Arthritis Rheum 1980; 23: 137–45.

14. Wolfe F. A reappraisal of HAQ disability in rheumatoid arthritis. Arthritis Rheum 2000; 43: 2751–61.

15. Drossaers-Bakker KW, Zwinderman AH, Vlieland TP et al. Long-term outcome in rheumatoid arthritis: a simple algorithm of baseline parameters can predict radiographic damage, disability, and disease course at 12-year follow up. Arthritis Care Res 2002; 47: 383–90.

16. Kirwan JR. Links between radiological change, disability, and pathology in rheumatoid arthritis. J Rheumatol 2001; 28: 881–6.

17. Mattey DL, Hassell AB, Dawes PT et al. Independent association of rheumatoid factor and the HLA-DRB1 shared epitope with radiographic outcome in rheumatoid arthritis. Arthritis Rheum 2001; 44: 1529–33.

18. Goronzy JJ, Matteson EL, Fulbright JW et al. Prognostic markers of radiographic progression in early rheumatoid arthritis. Arthritis Rheum 2004; 50: 43–54.

19. Vittecoq O, Pouplin S, Krzanowska K et al. Rheumatoid factor is the strongest predictor of radiological progression of rheumatoid arthritis in a three-year prospective study in community-recruited patients. Rheumatology (Oxford) 2003; 42: 939–46.

20. Bukhari M, Lunt M, Harrison BJ, Scott DG, Symmons DP, Silman AJ. Rheumatoid factor is the major predictor of increasing severity of radiographic erosions in rheumatoid arthritis: results from the Norfolk Arthritis Register Study, a large inception cohort. Arthritis Rheum 2002; 46: 906–12.

21. Nielen MM, van der Horst AR, van Schaardenburg D et al. Antibodies to citrullinated human fibrinogen (ACF) have diagnostic and prognostic value in early arthritis. Ann Rheum Dis 2005; 64: 1199–204.

22. Wakefield RJ, Gibbon WW, Conaghan PG et al. The value of sonography in the detection of bone erosions in patients with rheumatoid arthritis: a comparison with conventional radiography. Arthritis Rheum 2000; 43: 2762–70.

23. Skoumal M, Kolarz G, Klingler A. Serum levels of cartilage oligomeric matrix protein. A predicting factor and a valuable parameter for disease management in rheumatoid arthritis. Scand J Rheumatol 2003; 32: 156–61.

24. Radstake TR, Sweep FC, Welsing P et al. Correlation of rheumatoid arthritis severity with the genetic functional variants and circulating levels of macrophage migration inhibitory factor. Arthritis Rheum 2005; 52: 3020–9.

25. Taylor PC, Steuer A, Gruber J et al. Comparison of ultrasonographic assessment of synovitis and joint vascularity with radiographic evaluation in a randomized, placebo-controlled study of Infliximab therapy in early rheumatoid arthritis. Arthritis Rheum 2004; 50: 1107–16.

26. Drossaers-Bakker KW, de Buck M, van Zeben D, Zwinderman AH, Breedveld FC, Hazes JM. Long-term course and outcome of functional capacity in rheumatoid arthritis: the effects of disease activity and radiologic damage over time. Arthritis Rheum 1999; 42: 1854–60.

4 Goals of therapy

Overview
Other goals of treatment
Risk–benefit ratio of drug therapy

Overview

Over the last two decades, the goals of therapy in rheumatoid arthritis have been continually revised. There have been a number of reasons for this. In past decades, the treatment strategy was based on the premise that disease prognosis is generally favourable. However, careful studies of the natural history of rheumatoid arthritis clearly indicated that the majority of patients with a more aggressive disease evolution become clinically disabled within 20 years. For those with severe disease or extra-articular features, the mortality is equivalent to that of patients with three-vessel coronary artery disease or stage IV Hodgkin's lymphoma.[1] As a result, the notion that rheumatoid arthritis is a benign disease has been entirely discredited.

Historically, in the early stages of clinical presentation, non-steroidal anti-inflammatory drugs (NSAIDs) formed the mainstay of pharmacological intervention because of their effectiveness in terms of controlling certain symptoms and signs, and in the belief that their toxicity was relatively low compared to the so-called disease-modifying anti-rheumatic drugs (DMARDs) that were available 20 years or so ago. However, this paradigm too has been discredited, in part because of observations indicating that radiological evidence shows bone destruction takes place early in many patients and that NSAIDs have no benefit in terms of the destructive phase of rheumatoid

arthritis. Furthermore, the concept that NSAIDs have a relatively benign toxicity profile as compared with DMARDs has also been questioned, particularly in recent years.

There have been many other drivers towards changing the goals of therapy away from simply ameliorating symptoms of disease. These include a number of key studies indicating improved outcomes with optimal use of available oral DMARDs, either singly or in combination, with a clear demonstration that significant improvement in efficacy need not be at the expense of unacceptably high toxicity or tolerability problems. As a result, a strong trend has arisen towards much earlier use of DMARDs in the pharmacological management of disease. In the last decade, the advent of biological therapies, and in particular those targeting TNF-α, have further improved the expectation for magnitude of improvement in symptoms and signs of disease. As studies have been undertaken to determine the optimum use of biological therapies, it has become clear that a majority of patients benefit from a very significant inhibition of structural damage to joints of a magnitude not formerly seen with DMARDs alone. Furthermore, by means of strategies designed to suppress synovitis intensively, using either conventional DMARDs or biological therapies in combination with methotrexate, remission has become an achievable goal for a proportion of patients. Indeed, preliminary data from recent studies, to be discussed further in later chapters, suggest that biological-free remission may be achieved following an initial period of biological remission induction in the early phase of rheumatoid arthritis. As might be expected, with the demonstration of improved outcomes with respect to both symptoms and signs of disease as well as joint damage, for many patients preservation or improvement of functional status is also an achievable goal.

There is every reason to be optimistic about the outlook of patients presenting with rheumatoid arthritis at the present time. Twenty years ago, it could not be stated unequivocally that any of the available therapies halted the destructive process responsible for irreversible damage to cartilage, bone, and soft tissue. At that time, at best, the available therapies diminished the destruction modestly and inconsistently. In contrast, at present, although it cannot be unequivocally stated that cure of rheumatoid arthritis is possible, the outlook for most patients is favourable, although the current expectation is that the majority will be on long-term or life-long medication. The contemporary approach to management of rheumatoid arthritis, including pharmacological intervention, will be discussed in depth in following chapters.

Summary of goals of therapy

- Control of symptoms and signs

- Retardation or prevention of structural damage to joints

- Preservation and improvement in function

- Remission induction

Other goals of treatment

Other goals of treatment, closely aligned to the four domains listed above, include restoration and maintenance of a quality of life that permits the individual to pursue normal work, domestic, and social activity

---

To reduce the co-morbidity and increased mortality associated with both rheumatoid arthritis itself and with some treatment

---

It will be noted that the four primary goals listed above are closely aligned to the end-points used in the context of clinical trials. As pharmacological interventions suppress various inflammatory pathways responsible for the clinical expression of disease, it might also be said that normalisation of abnormal laboratory tests of inflammation and other markers of disease process, such as abnormal haematopoietic function, is a goal of therapy.

Risk–benefit ratio of drug therapy

The achievable goals of therapy need to be evaluated on an individual patient basis, and the rheumatologist must formulate an appropriate treatment plan to be discussed and agreed with the patient. In particular, it is absolutely necessary to optimise the gains of therapy while minimising the potential toxicities of drugs. Furthermore, the expense of biological agents in particular is such that it is necessary to operate within the health economic constraints of any given healthcare system. In practice, this may mean that certain therapies are only available when used within a setting of nationally agreed guidelines.

Reference

1. Pincus T, Callahan LF. What is the natural history of rheumatoid arthritis? *Rheum Dis Clin North Am* 1993; **19**: 123–51.

5 The multidisciplinary approach

Introduction
Education
Occupational therapy
Physiotherapy
Surgery
Nutrition and dietary therapy
Podiatry
Concluding remarks

Introduction

It is important to recognise that pharmacological intervention represents only one aspect of the management plan for rheumatoid arthritis at any given stage of disease, irrespective of its severity. Other important aspects of the total management plan include patient education and, where necessary, psychological and employment counselling. The optimum quality of life and functioning can be supported by a realistic evaluation of the most appropriate level of rest and exercise, and coping with activities of daily living. In this respect, appropriate access to splints, aids, and adaptations can help preserve function and maintain independence and mobility. Counselling and information about access to social and financial benefits is also of great importance. Appropriate comfortable footwear and proper care of the feet, particularly in those patients with established deformities, can help maintain mobility and comfort. Surgical treatment may also play an essential role in relieving intractable pain and may help restore physical functioning and mobility lost as a result of mechanical damage to joints and associated structures. Surgery may

also be invaluable in the treatment of secondary complications of joint disease, such as peripheral nerve entrapment at the wrist or elbow, and cervical cord compression in relation to instability of the cervical spine.

The success of pharmacological intervention requires that the patient, where possible, is involved in the reasoning behind prescribing a particular therapy and gives informed consent to the treatment regimen. Family members and carers will also wish to be involved in this process and to have a thorough understanding of the potential benefits and risks of treatment as well as appropriate drug monitoring and other means of reducing the risk of any toxicity. Because rheumatoid arthritis is a chronic disease, the majority of patients will have a long-term relationship with their health care providers. Therefore, a holistic approach to patient care is dependent on multidisciplinary teamwork and co-ordination of patient care between physicians in primary and secondary care settings, and a number of other key healthcare professionals, including specialist nurses, physiotherapists, occupational therapists, podiatrists, social workers, pharmacists, and surgeons.

Education

All members of the multidisciplinary team are likely to be involved in patient education. The purpose of this is to help the patient and, where appropriate, their families, friends, colleagues, and carers, to understand the nature of rheumatoid arthritis better and thus to cope with the condition as well as possible. Most patients cope much better if they understand their condition and have realistic expectations of the benefits and disadvantages of the various treatment interventions, including drug therapies. With the help of their doctors and other healthcare workers, both short- and long-term management plans can be formulated, and the role of standard and alternative therapies discussed. Education is an on-going process and there is only a certain amount of information that the patient is able to take in on the first few visits. It is important that the newly presenting patient is aware that rheumatoid arthritis is not (currently) a curable condition but that, nonetheless, with optimum therapy and regular assessment, the outlook has become greatly improved in recent years. A number of excellent patient education leaflets are available such as those distributed by the Arthritis Research Campaign.

Educational interventions which include a psychobehavioural component in addition to providing information alone can lead to better outcomes with respect to pain relief, joint protection, and functional disability. However, they have the disadvantage of being labour-intensive and, in general, are only available where there is a sizable multidisciplinary team in a large secondary care setting.[1,2] A good education programme can also do much to improve self-esteem for patients and to allow them to feel that they have control over their illness. It is also important for relatives and carers to understand the patient's condition and needs.

Education is not only important for the patient but also for other members of the multidisciplinary team. This is particularly true for primary care practitioners, who are often the first port of call for patients in times of need. Education is particularly important in primary care because the treatment paradigm for rheumatoid arthritis has changed at a rapid pace, with concomitant improvement in patient outcomes and higher expectations of therapeutic intervention. It has also become clear that much potential toxicity associated with pharmacological intervention is preventable with appropriate drug monitoring programmes. There are various models on which such programmes can be set up, many of which involve shared care between primary and secondary practitioners. It is, therefore, essential that there is a good dialogue between primary and secondary care practitioners and the patients. Many hospital centres will have close relationships with their primary care

partners, with regular educational programmes to explain changing principles in the treatment of rheumatoid arthritis and the most appropriate role of primary care practitioners in ensuring optimum drug safety. Similarly, secondary care practitioners need to be educated by their primary care colleagues regarding their needs and expectations for patients referred.

Occupational therapy

Occupational therapists look at the function of the patient in the context of their disability. They provide joint protection advice and play a major role in patient education. They have expertise in assessing joint function and provide various aids and adaptations as required to help improve function and limit discomfort during a particular activity. For example, for patients with advanced arthritis and poor hand function, the provision of simple handle grips for cutlery may make it considerably easier for them to feed themselves. Similarly, devices to remove lids from bottles or turn on taps or perform many other everyday activities which most able-bodied people take for granted can make a considerable difference to the quality of life for a patient with rheumatoid arthritis, and may even permit a patient with advanced deformities to maintain a level of independence that would not be possible otherwise.

Occupational therapists also assess patients with a view to the provision of splints. Resting splints are used during acute joint exacerbations. Afterwards, serial splints can be customised to the particular shape of a patient's joint and used with semi-static resting splints, progressing to dynamic splints as required. Rest splinting of involved joints can help to reduce pain and improve function, and finger splinting may help to reduce deformities and preserve or even improve hand function.

The occupational therapist may also ask the patient about hobbies and recreational activities when making an assessment. They will enquire about the patient's ability to undertake personal hygiene, grooming, eating, drinking, dressing, getting in and out of bed, and everyday activities such as driving, cleaning, cooking, shopping, and work-related activities. The occupational therapist will also give the patient an opportunity to discuss issues related to personal relationships and intimacy if they wish to. By looking at these different spheres of activity within the patient's life, the occupational therapist will suggest strategies to overcome limitations imposed by joint inflammation and mechanical problems. They will also teach patients to conserve energy by use of joint protection techniques. Some of the principles of joint rest and protection include: (i) conservation of energy by promoting an appropriate balance between work and rest; (ii) good use of body mechanics; (iii) making arrangements to sit rather than stand while working, if possible; and (iv) to use larger joints where possible. Advice about lifting will also be given, including the use of two hands rather than one, sliding objects instead of lifting them, and avoiding a tight grip or twisting motion of the hands where possible. Patients may be advised to take note of any pain associated with their arthritis and to regard it as a signal not to exceed a certain level of activity with respect to the painful area.

Physiotherapy

The physiotherapist (or physical therapist) plays a role in assessing function and activity and implementing a programme to help pain relief initially and rehabilitation in the longer term. Acute management may include resting or immobilising acutely inflamed joints and maintaining the range of joint movement by active movement and passive stretching exercises. Local application of heat or cold may provide symptomatic relief to soft tissues and some physiotherapy departments will also use laser or ultrasound treatments for this purpose.

Patients with rheumatoid arthritis often stop using their inflamed joints because of pain and stiffness. Resting an acutely inflamed joint may be entirely appropriate in the short-term, but

prolonged inactivity can lead to rapid loss of muscle strength with accompanying loss of joint motion and ultimately contractions. As good muscle bulk and tone predominantly determine joint stability, weakness of muscles can decrease stability and thus further exacerbate fatigue associated with arthritis. A regular exercise programme tailored to the needs of the individual patient can help to prevent and even reverse such effects. A physiotherapist has expertise in recommending different kinds of exercise that may be beneficial. These include range-of-motion exercises, to preserve and restore joint movement, various isometric, isotonic, or isokinetic exercises designed to increase muscle strength, or exercises to increase stamina and endurance. Examples of the latter include walking, swimming, and cycling. It is best to select an exercise that is within the capabilities of the individual patient and also one that will be enjoyed and, therefore, more likely to be undertaken regularly.

Although there are relatively few controlled studies illustrating the benefits of physical therapy in the way that studies are undertaken to investigate the effectiveness of pharmacological intervention, it is nonetheless well established that, over the short-term, regular aerobic exercise improves muscle function, joint stability, aerobic capacity, and overall physical functioning with improved pain control without exacerbating the underlying arthritic condition. Furthermore, aerobic weight-bearing exercise can help to prevent the bone loss that is associated with long-term steroid treatment.

Physiotherapists may also recommend and oversee a course of hydrotherapy, a course of exercises undertaken in a warm pool. This can be a very valuable way of mobilising joints and provides exercise in a non-impact, buoyant environment, with a view to restoring muscle tone and power. As joints become less inflamed and muscle strength improves, movement is encouraged with active exercises against progressive resistance.

Where appropriate, physiotherapists will assess the patient's gait and, in particular, the appropriateness of a walking aid such as a stick. A large variety of walking stick designs are available, and the most effective will be one of a length measured for the exact needs of an individual patient and with a handgrip that allows optimum use, depending on the upper limb, hand, and wrist involvement of the arthritis.

Surgery

The aims of surgical intervention are to relieve pain and, where possible, to restore function. Indications for urgent surgical treatment include ruptured tendons, and compression of nerves and spinal cord. Septic arthritis may also require urgent surgical intervention, although many cases can be treated as a medical emergency.

The patient needs to be involved in decisions regarding possible surgical treatments, and must have an understanding of the potential range of benefits and adverse effects that might occur. Functional restriction in any given joint can be thought of in terms of two components – inflammatory and mechanical. The goal of medical treatment is to suppress the inflammatory component as optimally as possible. Where synovitis is refractory to medical treatment, however, surgical intervention may be necessary to remove inflammatory tissue in the form of synovectomy. Such procedures may retard the rate of damage to a given joint over a short time period but, in general, do not alter the final outcome. For this reason, surgical synovectomy is less commonly undertaken than it used to be. It is desirable to suppress synovitis optimally before undertaking surgery to ensure the most favourable outcome. However, it should also be remembered that infection is always one of the most feared risks of joint surgery; for this reason, many orthopaedic surgeons would prefer that potent immunosuppressive therapy, in particular biological treatments, are discontinued for a short peri-operative period. There is data to suggest that there is no need to discontinue disease-modifying anti-rheumatic drugs (DMARDs) for long periods prior to surgery but, as yet, there is no consensus as to the best timing for cessation of biological therapies prior to a given surgical procedure, or for their re-instatement afterwards. As a general rule, it is best to ensure that wound healing has taken place satisfactorily without any evidence of infection before recommencing a biological therapy if it has been stopped prior to surgery.

Co-ordination between the rheumatologists and orthopaedic surgeon is also very helpful when considering the timing and sequence of procedures when multiple surgeries are contemplated. The patient needs to be involved at every stage of the decision-making process where possible. For example, forefoot arthroplasty, if indicated, should usually precede knee or hip arthroplasty to minimise the risk of infection.

The range of surgical procedures available is now very considerable, and the enormous beneficial impact of hip and knee arthroplasties in improving the quality of life for innumerable patients cannot be under-estimated. Corrective surgical procedures that may be required include: (i) cervical fusion for subluxation; (ii) replacement arthroplasties; and (iii) excision arthroplasties or arthrodesis.

Nutrition and dietary therapy

Active rheumatoid arthritis may be accompanied by a loss of appetite and, in severe cases, rheumatoid-associated cachexia. For more frail patients with poor mobility, inadequate dietary intake may represent a problem. As part of a management plan that may also involve a dietician, advice should be given to ensure that the patient's diet comprises an adequate amount of calories and appropriate nutrients. However, if the patient is overweight and particularly if obese, weight loss should be recommended to reduce the burden on large weight-bearing joints.

Much research indicates that chronic inflammation associated with rheumatoid arthritis is linked with a significant rise in cardiovascular risk. It is, therefore, appropriate to check blood cholesterol levels and if need be for a dietician to recommend an appropriate diet and life-style to reduce serum cholesterol. If need be, drug therapy may also be necessary. Similarly, patients who smoke should be counselled to discontinue if possible, but even reducing cigarette consumption can be helpful.

Numerous diets have been proposed to benefit patients with arthritis, and there is much popular literature extolling the virtues of one particular diet or another. However, there is little scientific evidence to support strongly that any particular diet has a universally beneficial outcome. This does not mean that a diet will not have a value for a particular patient and there is much to be said for encouraging patients to try a diet as part of their effort to take control of their own condition. Omega-3-rich oils have a modest benefit in terms of arthritis pain and joint swelling; therefore, fish oil supplements and some plant oils, such as flax seed and borage seed oil, may be of value, or a diet enriched in oily fish. Similarly, vegetable intake is to be encouraged and some dieticians will recommend a reduction in red meat. Certain patients may report that their arthritis is aggravated by particular foods; if this is so, then it is reasonable to advise avoidance in individual cases.

Podiatry

Rheumatoid arthritis commonly involves the feet and, as such, can potentially cause major limitations to mobility. Podiatrists take a specialist interest in foot health. They can give advice about local redistribution of loading to prevent the formation of calluses, and to treat such lesions appropriately when they do arise. Furthermore, podiatrists may provide specialised footwear customised to the needs of the individual and also customised orthoses and insoles to improve foot and toe posture and function. Provision of general foot care is very important, with a view to preventing local infection and maintaining function.

Concluding remarks

The importance of the role of the multidisciplinary team should be considered as part of good practice. All patients with early rheumatoid arthritis should have access to a range of health professionals, including the nurse specialist, physiotherapist, occupational therapist, dietician, podiatrist, pharmacist, and social worker as required. The primary care physicians and secondary care rheumatologists will also be seen on a regular basis. All members of this multidisciplinary team in both primary and secondary care settings have an important role to play in patient education and in ensuring best possible outcomes.

References

1. Superio-Cabuslay E, Ward MM, Lorig KR. Patient education interventions in osteoarthritis and rheumatoid arthritis: a meta-analytic comparison with nonsteroidal antiinflammatory drug treatment. *Arthritis Care Res* 1996; **9**: 292–301.

2. Evers AW, Kraaimaat FW, Geenen R, Bijlsma JW. Psychosocial predictors of functional change in recently diagnosed rheumatoid arthritis patients. *Behav Res Ther* 1998; **36**: 179–93.

6 Pharmacotherapeutics in rheumatoid arthritis

Introduction
Non-steroidal anti-inflammatory drugs
  (NSAIDs)
Corticosteroids
Disease-modifying anti-rheumatic
  drugs (DMARDs)
Drug treatment during pregnancy
Combination non-biological DMARD
  therapy
Step-up clinical trial strategies
Step-down combination DMARD
  strategies
Summary

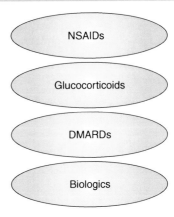

Figure 6.1
Pharmacotherapeutics in rheumatoid arthritis.

Introduction

Drug therapy for rheumatoid arthritis can usefully be thought of as falling into one of four categories of therapeutics (Fig. 6.1) – non-steroidal anti-inflammatory drugs (NSAIDs), glucocorticoids, disease-modifying anti-rheumatic drugs (DMARDs), and biological therapies. Patients will not necessarily need to be exposed to drugs from each of these categories during the course of their disease. Selection and optimisation of a drug regimen for any given individual is best advised by a secondary care specialist and, where possible, involving the patient in the decision-making process. It is also important for specialist rheumatologists to work in close partnership with their primary care colleagues in order to minimise any drug toxicities and maximise the benefits of therapy.

The first three of these four drug categories will be discussed in the present chapter. Biological therapies will be introduced and discussed in detail in chapters to follow.

Non-steroidal anti-inflammatory drugs (NSAIDs)

NSAIDs are weak organic acids that bind avidly to serum proteins. For the majority, when in the acidic environment of the stomach, they are in the non-ionised form but, in some cases, this non-ionised form is associated with local mucosal damage. However, a beneficial property of acidic NSAIDs is that they may accumulate preferentially in inflamed joints and persist there longer than would be predicted on the basis of their serum half-life.

NSAIDs have both analgesic and anti-inflammatory properties but only for certain inflammatory pathways. Thus they give rise to effective symptom control in a proportion of rheumatoid arthritis patients but have **no effect** on disease progression.

Practice point

NSAIDs have analgesic and anti-inflammatory properties. They give rise to effective symptom control in a proportion of rheumatoid arthritis patients, but have **no effect** on disease progression.

The medicinal use of willow bark for treatment of pain and fever has been recorded since ancient times. Willow bark and other plants contain salicylates, in which the active principle, salicylin, forms the basis of salicylic acid. Acetylsalicylate, better known as aspirin, was first synthesised in 1853 but was not used until the late 19th century. Indomethacin was not introduced until over a century later, in 1965, and inhibition of cyclo-oxygenase with consequential reduction in prostaglandin synthesis, a major mechanism of action, was described by John Vane in 1971 (Fig. 6.2). The Nobel Prize was awarded for this discovery. Further advances in the field were made in the 1990s, when it was discovered that there is more than one cyclo-oxygenase enzyme.

Mechanism of action of NSAIDs

The major mechanism of action of NSAIDs is thought to be inhibition of cyclo-oxygenase, an enzyme that catalyzes the conversion of arachidonic acid, a product of cell membrane breakdown, into prostaglandins. There are many different members of the prostaglandin family, some of which contribute to pathological features of inflammation, including pain, fever, and swelling. Joint stiffness may also be greatly improved by prostaglandin inhibition. However, other prostaglandins are required for

normal physiological processes including the support of renal function, platelet function, and protection of gastric mucosa. As a consequence, use of NSAIDs that inhibit prostaglandins associated with physiological functioning may result in various toxicities. These will be discussed below.

Following the original discovery that NSAIDs inhibited cyclo-oxygenase, it became clear that, in fact, there are at least two isoforms of the enzyme, cyclo-oxygenase one (COX-1) and cyclo-oxygenase two (COX-2). Both enzymes have a molecular weight of 70 kDa but are encoded by different genes. COX-1, encoded on chromosome 9, is thought to be constitutively expressed. The gene is a so-called 'housekeeping gene' producing a continuously transcribed, stable message. The protein is expressed in the stomach, intestine, kidneys, and platelets. COX-2, on the other hand, is encoded by chromosome 1. In contrast to COX-1, COX-2 is cytokine-inducible and is thought to be responsible for many of the undesirable features of inflammation that occur in pathological states such as rheumatoid arthritis. However, COX-2 is also constitutively expressed in the kidney and brain. The theoretical importance of the discovery of COX-2 was the hope that many of the commoner toxicities associated with COX-1 inhibition, in

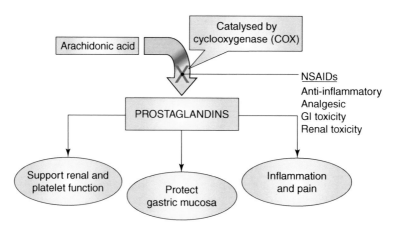

Figure 6.2
Initial concept for mechanism of action of NSAIDs.

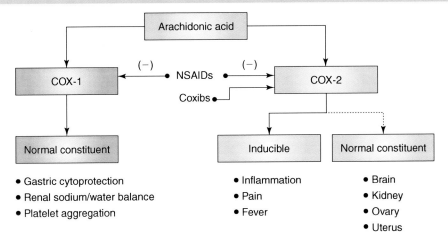

Figure 6.3
Different functions of the COX-1 and COX-2 enzymes.

particular gastric side-effects, might be obviated by targeting the COX-2 enzyme (Fig. 6.3).

Although some NSAIDs are almost entirely specific for blockade of the COX-1 enzyme, and others almost entirely specific for COX-2, many will inhibit both enzymes to a varying degree. Thus, indomethacin and naproxyn may be said to inhibit the COX-1 enzyme selectively, nabumetone, meloxicam, and etodolac selectively inhibit the COX-2 enzyme, whereas etoricoxib and lumeracoxib specifically inhibit COX-2.

Efficacy of NSAIDs

Clinical trials and experience both suggest that COX-2 inhibitors have very similar efficacy to that of traditional NSAIDs. There are no clear-cut relationships between degree of cyclo-oxygenase inhibition and efficacy for symptoms and signs of disease, and in general, there are poor correlations between plasma level of a given drug and efficacy, with the notable exception of salicylates. It is also of note that there are clear individual variations in response to a given NSAID. In practice, therefore, it may be necessary to have a therapeutic trial of two or three different NSAIDs sequentially in order to determine the most efficacious and best tolerated for a given individual. NSAIDs have an analgesic potency equivalent to that of narcotics in therapeutic doses in acute pain. Inhibition of prostaglandins in the central nervous system has an anti-pyretic effect and anti-inflammatory benefits include reduced swelling and stiffness. NSAIDs with the capability of inhibiting the COX-1 enzyme have an anti-platelet effect, decreasing platelet aggregation by prevention of thromboxin A_2 production.

Toxicity of NSAIDs

Adverse events commonly associated with NSAIDs that predominantly inhibit the COX-1 enzyme include numerous upper gastrointestinal effects. These include dyspepsia, erosion, gastrointestinal bleeding with secondary anaemia, or even peptic ulceration with bleeding or perforation. Furthermore, anti-platelet effects may contribute to blood loss. Some degree of gastrointestinal intolerance is a common problem with traditional NSAIDs. In one study of pooled data on the incidence of nausea, abdominal pain, and dyspepsia from eight controlled osteoarthritis and rheumatoid arthritis trials of at least 12 weeks' duration, over 12% of patients experienced some form of gastrointestinal distress.[1] Up to 10% of patients taking NSAIDs in the long term may experience gastric ulceration:[2] in some series, over 1% of patients taking traditional NSAIDs may require hospitalisation for an upper gastrointestinal emergency.[3]

It is important to appreciate that gastrointestinal side-effects may be devoid of any warning symptoms. In a large study of 1921 patients, 81% had no premonitory symptoms prior to a serious NSAID-associated gastrointestinal event such as bleeding, perforation, or gastric outlet obstruction.[4]

Predictive factors for NSAID-induced gastroduodenal ulcer disease include age over 60 years, past history of peptic ulcer disease, with or without NSAIDs, and higher NSAID dosages. Other factors include previous use of antacids, H2-blockers, or proton-pump inhibitors, gastrointestinal symptoms, anti-coagulant therapy, concomitant steroid usage, tobacco and/or alcohol use and a history of abdominal pain of uncertain aetiology. Existing *Helicobacter pylori* infection may also predispose toward NSAID-induced complications.

Various steps can be taken to reduce the likelihood of gastrointestinal toxicity in patients treated with traditional NSAIDs to inhibit the COX-1 enzymes. It is always necessary to reconsider whether an NSAID is really appropriate at all. If pain is the predominant symptom, then it may be more appropriate to use a plain analgesic. However, NSAIDs can be extremely helpful and are appropriate for those patients with inflammatory features including marked stiffness. In such cases, it is wise to use the lowest effective dose of NSAID possible. In high-risk patients, proton-pump inhibitors may be co-prescribed, and there is good evidence that they are protective against the ulcer-inducing effect of traditional NSAIDs. An alternative approach is to prescribe a COX-2 selective or specific NSAID. When COX-2 inhibitors were first developed, it was hoped

that they would have all the benefits of an NSAID, without the associated toxicities. New clinical trial data indicate that COX-2 inhibitors are significantly less gastrotoxic than traditional NSAID comparators but it is not the case that they are free of tolerability problems and they may still cause dyspepsia. COX-2 inhibitors became very widely used in the early years of the new millennium; however, with increased usage, it became clear that certain of these drugs were associated with other toxicities, most notably cardiovascular complications as discussed below.

Practice point

It is always necessary to reconsider whether an NSAID is really the most appropriate medication to prescribe. If pain is the predominant symptom, then it may be better to use a plain analgesic.

Other side-effects of NSAIDs include hepatotoxicity. NSAIDs are cleared predominantly by hepatic metabolism, with the production of inactive metabolites that are excreted in the urine. Elevation of liver enzymes may occur with all NSAIDs; transaminase levels, in particular, are commonly raised and this may particularly cause concern for patients on regular drug monitoring for methotrexate therapy. More serious hepatitis or cholestasis are much rarer complications.

In hypovolaemic states and renal insufficiency, prostaglandins are required to maintain adequate glomerular flow. Inhibitors of both COX-1 and COX-2 may have nephrotoxic side-effects. These include reduced glomerular filtration, increased serum creatinine, increased sodium retention and blood volume (which makes NSAIDs relatively contra-indicated in patients with congestive cardiac failure), hyperkalaemia, or hyponatraemia. Other uncommon toxicities include capillary necrosis and interstitial nephritis. For these reasons, NSAIDs are relatively contra-indicated in patients with mild renal impairment. However, the non-acetylated salicylates are poor prostaglandin inhibitors and may have fewer detrimental effects on glomerular filtration. Sulindac is a pro-drug that is converted in the body to an active form, sulindac sulphide. It is converted back into sulindac in the kidney, diminishing the potential nephrotoxic effect of prostaglandin inhibition in this organ. Although the COX-2 enzyme is cytokine-inducible to a greater extent than COX-1, COX-2 is expressed in the glomeruli and renal vasculature.

Hypertension is a common complication of NSAID use. Blood pressure thus requires monitoring and, if need be, treating. However, fewer than 1% of patients need to withdraw from NSAID therapy for this reason.

Other complications of NSAIDs include tinnitus associated with salicylates. Other central nervous system effects include headaches, dizziness, and poor concentration.

Following the rapid uptake of COX-2 inhibitors after their introduction, a number of cardiovascular complications came to light. In the VIGOR study, designed to compare the risk of developing a clinical upper gastrointestinal event in rheumatoid patients treated with rofecoxib at a dose of 50 mg once daily, compared with naproxyn 500 mg twice daily, it emerged that there was a greater risk of myocardial infarction in the rofecoxib-treated patients than the naproxyn-treated patients. At first, this was thought to reflect a relative cardioprotective effect of naproxyn mediated through its anti-platelet action; rofecoxib, as a COX-2-specific drug, by definition has no anti-platelet effect.[5] In the CLASS study, the incidence of ulcer complications was compared in a cohort of patients with either osteoarthritis or rheumatoid arthritis randomised to receive treatment with celecoxib at a dose of 400 mg b.d., diclofenac 75 mg. b.d., or ibuprofen 800 mg t.d.s. In this study, the risk of myocardial infarction was similar in the celecoxib and ibuprofen groups, although there was a trend to a higher risk of myocardial infarction for patients taking celecoxib versus those on diclofenac.[6] Rofecoxib was subsequently withdrawn from the global market

in September 2004, following preliminary findings from the APPROVe (adenomatous polyp prevention) trial. In this study, there were 1.5 thrombotic events per 100 patient-years in rofecoxib-treated patients versus 0.78 events per 100 patient-years after 18 months of treatment.[7] Another COX-2-specific inhibitor, valdecoxib, was withdrawn following the finding of an increased incidence of cardiovascular events after coronary artery bypass grafting.[8] There are other re-assuring safety data regarding cardiovascular toxicity in a population of osteoarthritis patients treated with either etoricoxib or diclofenac sodium. It is not entirely clear why, in certain diseases, some COX-2 inhibitors appear to cause more thombotic events than traditional NSAIDs with prolonged use. However, abnormal blood vessels require COX-2 to produce prostaglandin I-2 (prostacyclin), which is anti-thrombotic. The unaffected COX-2 enzyme, which is constitutively expressed, is necessary for production of thromboxane A_2, which is a potent platelet inhibitor. It is, therefore, conceivable that COX-2 inhibition may favour a pro-thrombotic environment in certain circumstances.

Summary

NSAIDs have been available for a particularly long time and are widely prescribed. There is no doubt that many patients with rheumatoid arthritis will derive considerable symptomatic benefit from the use of these drugs. However, the view that they have little associated toxicity is unfounded and some members of the newer generation of COX-2 inhibitors are also associated with cardiovascular risk. Therefore, NSAIDs must be used with care, with a view to maximising benefits and minimising any toxicities, as is the case with any drug. Particular caution must be exercised in elderly patients with rheumatoid arthritis. The most important question to ask before prescribing an NSAID is whether such a drug is actually required or whether a plain analgesic will suffice. Where prescription of an NSAID is justified in the elderly patient, it is reasonable to start at the lowest dose and to follow-up closely with a view to monitoring therapeutic benefit and any toxicity or tolerability problems. Good communication between primary and secondary care practitioners when prescribing such drugs is very helpful in ensuring the best quality monitoring.

Corticosteroids

The Nobel Prize was awarded in 1950 to Hench and Kendall for the discovery of corticosteroids in 1949. These drugs potently suppress aspects of inflammation and have immunosuppressive properties. When first discovered, they were hailed as miracle drugs because of their potency in certain previously untreatable disorders. However, since that time, growing appreciation of the associated toxicities has limited their use. Nonetheless, corticosteroids remain widely used in the treatment of rheumatoid arthritis and may be administered by a number of different routes, both oral and parenteral.

Mechanism of action of corticosteroids

Corticosteroids exert anti-inflammatory and immunosuppressive effects through numerous mechanisms. Corticosteroids bind an intracellular cytoplasmic receptor which promotes nuclear translocation and binding to steroid response elements in the promoters of genes. For example, transcriptional activation of the inhibitor of kappa B (IκBα gene) inhibits the nuclear transcription factor NF-κB. Corticosteroids also interfere with the activity of the transcription factors Ap-1 and NF-AT. In the case of Ap-1, corticosteroids stoichiometrically interfere with Ap-1 binding with the steroid receptor. Transcriptional activation of IκB promotes down-regulation of a number of key pro-inflammatory pathways, including adhesion molecule expression and secretion of pro-inflammatory cytokines such as IL-1 and TNF-α. Consequences include reduced leukocyte margination and inflammatory cell recruitment from the vascular compartment to the involved tissues. There is also inhibition of granulocyte and macrophage phagocytosis and

enzyme release, induction of lipocortin-1, with consequent inhibition of phospholipase A-II, which, in turn, decreases arachidonic acid synthesis and thereby reduces prostaglandin and leukotriene production. In common with some NSAIDs, corticosteroids also inhibit the COX-2 enzyme. Other mechanisms of action include reduced T-cell proliferation, together with IL-2 secretion, and promotion of lymphocyte apoptosis.

Potential benefits of corticosteroids in rheumatoid arthritis

Corticosteroids rapidly and potently suppress inflammatory processes and have efficacy for systemic and local components of inflammation in rheumatoid arthritis. Corticosteroids can be used as a 'bridging' therapy when a more slowly acting oral DMARD is initiated so that rapid suppression of synovitis can be achieved before the slower benefits of the DMARD are expressed. The dose of steroid can subsequently be tapered. Because of their potency, corticosteroids have a place in treatment of many of the extra-articular complications of rheumatoid arthritis, including vasculitis, and in those patients with systemic features of disease such as rheumatoid cachexia and pyrexia. However, the usefulness of corticosteroids is significantly limited by potentially serious toxicities. Many of these complications can be minimised by use of appropriate dosing regimens and mode of administration and, where appropriate, concomitant administration of bisphosphonates as prophylaxis for steroid-induced osteoporosis.

Mode of administration of corticosteroids

In addition to oral administration, corticosteroids can be given parenterally by the intramuscular or intravenous routes or as intrasynovial therapy by needle injection into joints, bursae, or tendon sheaths. Intrasynovial corticosteroid injections alleviate inflammation in a particular joint, bursa, or tendon sheath, and avoid some of the complications of regular systemic therapy. This approach is particularly useful where one or a few sites remain refractory to DMARD therapy. The appropriate dose will depend on the size of the joint, degree of inflammation, and concentration of corticosteroid used. Fluorinated corticosteroids have the potential complication of subcutaneous fat atrophy and are best avoided in injection of more superficial sites.

Where joint fluids are present, they should be aspirated prior to steroid injection. When expertly administered, intrasynovial steroid injections can be very beneficial. However, repeated injections to the same site may be detrimental by accelerating cartilage breakdown or weakening a tendon. A minimum of 4–6 weeks between injections is desirable; in the case of weight-bearing joints, injection should not be performed more frequently than every 6–12 weeks. In general, it is best not to inject the same joint or tendon sheath more than three times in a year.

Skin and subcutaneous tissues can be anaesthetised with local anaesthetics using a fine needle prior to steroid injection; alternatively, anaesthetic preparations can be safely mixed with corticosteroid prior to injection.

Intramuscular, long-acting steroid can be used as a bridging therapy and treatment for flare of rheumatoid disease activity. A long-acting preparation is most appropriate, such as depomedrone, used at a dose of 120–160 mg.

Adverse consequences of corticosteroid therapy

Unfortunately, despite their rapid onset of action and many anti-inflammatory benefits, steroid administration by any route has a number of potential complications, many of which are serious. Adverse events associated with corticosteroids in general include the following:

- glucose intolerance
- osteoporosis
- osteonecrosis
- cataract formation
- thinning of the skin
- easy bruising
- delayed wound repair
- striae
- peptic ulceration (particularly when used in conjunction with COX-1 selected or specific NSAIDs)
- suppression of the hypothalamic–pituitary–adrenal axis
- depressed hormone levels, including TSH, testosterone, FSH, and LH
- growth suppression in children
- obesity
- hirsutism
- abnormal menstruation
- mental disturbance
- muscle weakness
- infection.

Corticosteroid injections may be complicated by infection, with an occurrence rate documented at about 1:50,000 injections in many series. Other complications include skin hypopigmentation (particularly noticeable in patients of darker skinned races), subcutaneous tissue atrophy, tendon rupture, osteonecrosis, and steroid crystal-induced post-injection flare (particularly following injection of the elbow joint). Post-injection flares occur in about 2% of injections and manifest within 6–18 hours following an injection, in contrast to a septic complication, which is generally slower to become apparent. Treatment of post-injection flare is with NSAIDs, analgesia, and local ice, following which the condition self-limits rapidly. However, when there is doubt as to the diagnosis, a joint must be aspirated to exclude infection. The aspirate will often reveal intracellular steroid crystals.

There are a number of relative and absolute contra-indications to intrasynovial corticosteroid injections. These include peri-articular or articular sepsis, bacteraemia, intra-articular fracture, bleeding diathesis, and lack of response to previous injections.

Exogenous corticosteroid administration suppresses ACTH production from the pituitary gland, and is the most common cause of adrenal insufficiency. Patients treated with ≥ 20 mg of prednisolone a day for over a month are likely to have suppression of the hypothalamic–pituitary–adrenal axis, as are those treated with 3–5 mg daily for more than a year. The implications of this suppression are that such patients are unable to respond naturally with a rise in cortisol output in response to physiological stresses such as infection, surgery, or trauma. In the case of patients for whom a short course of corticosteroids is clinically indicated, taking the medication early in the morning may minimise the suppressive effect on the hypothalamic–pituitary–adrenal axis because cortisol secretion peaks in the morning as part of a natural diurnal variation in production. However, the timing of dosing is probably less important for patients on long-term corticosteroid treatment.

It may take many months for the hypothalamic–pituitary–adrenal axis to recover after cessation of corticosteroid therapy, in particular for restoration of the normal adrenal response to ACTH. Steroid withdrawal syndrome may accompany rapid tapering or cessation of corticosteroid dose, and this may include confusion, arthralgia, and myalgia.

Steps to avoid corticosteroid-associated complications

Where possible, an appropriate history and examination should be undertaken to ensure that the patient does not have an underlying chronic infection. It is useful to obtain a baseline (random or even fasting) glucose level prior to institution of therapy, with subsequent periodic monitoring of blood and urine glucose.

Corticosteroids may be gastrotoxic in their own right and exacerbate the gastric toxicity associated with NSAIDs. A careful history for symptoms and risk factors for peptic ulceration needs to be taken and for patients at risk, co-prescription of a proton-pump inhibitor should

be considered. As in the case of NSAIDs, corticosteroids may exacerbate pre-existing hypertension and peripheral oedema, both of which need to be monitored throughout a course of therapy.

Osteoporosis is a particularly common complication of long-term steroid therapy, particularly at prednisolone doses in excess of 5 mg once daily. A baseline DEXA scan is helpful in assessing the risk of steroid-induced osteoporosis; for those patients on long-term therapy, follow-up DEXA scans will be required. Prophylaxis for corticosteroid-induced osteoporosis includes prescription of calcium to achieve a minimum intake of 1500 mg/day, together with vitamin D at a minimum dose of 400 IU/day. For those patients expected to be taking prednisolone at a dose in excess of 5 mg daily for more than 3 months, there is now a good evidence base to support the prophylactic use of a bisphosphonate for prevention of corticosteroid-induced osteoporosis.

Disease-modifying anti-rheumatic drugs (DMARDs)

Untreated, rheumatoid arthritis is a systemic inflammatory condition with its predominant expression in joints, and is characterised by an inflammatory joint disease that causes a variable degree of tissue destruction. Joint damage is cumulative over time and the rate of destruction is very variable between patients. The term disease-modifying anti-rheumatic drug or DMARD refers to a category of pharmacological agents that has some ability to retard the rate of structural joint damage. This property distinguishes DMARDs from NSAIDs, which improve certain features of inflammation, but have no capability to modify the rate of structural damage to joints in human disease, although they may do so in animal models. The term DMARD has also been applied to drugs that result in sustained improvement in physical function or a decrease in inflammatory synovitis.

Currently available drugs for the treatment of rheumatoid arthritis that are included within the category of DMARDs include methotrexate, sulphasalazine, hydroxychloroquine, leflunomide, gold (which is available as both intramuscular and oral preparations), and D-penicillamine.

It has become clear in recent years that the best outcomes in the management of rheumatoid arthritis are achieved when DMARD therapy is used optimally and as early as possible. Patients meeting classification criteria for rheumatoid arthritis will almost invariably require DMARD therapy, and there is emerging evidence to suggest that outcomes can be improved maximally if treatment is initiated at very early time-points, when patients still have an undifferentiated early inflammatory arthritis, prior to meeting classification criteria. Having said this, it must be accepted that a proportion of patients with undifferentiated, early inflammatory arthritis will have self-limiting disease, which emphasises the need for better diagnostic and prognostic markers that will be informative for management of early arthritis on an individual patient basis.

The concept of a 'window of opportunity' to achieve optimum responses to drug therapy following symptom onset in the early phase of disease will be discussed at length in Chapter 8.

Most DMARDs used in pharmacological management of rheumatoid arthritis need to be taken for 8 weeks or more before any significant symptomatic benefit is apparent, and it may take many months before a maximal response is achieved. It is very important that patients are aware of this, in order that they remain compliant with therapy, particularly if there are some initial tolerability problems such as nausea. All members of the multidisciplinary care team have a role in emphasising the importance of drug compliance and the reasons for prescribing DMARD therapy.

NSAIDs, corticosteroids, and biologics, particularly those targeting TNF-α, are associated with more rapid symptomatic benefits. Corticosteroids may be used as a bridging therapy, by orally administered drug or by means of intramuscular administration of a long-acting steroid such as depomedrone, in order to give a prescribed conventional DMARD a chance to work.

Methotrexate

Methotrexate is widely considered to have the best efficacy to toxicity ratio of the DMARDs. A higher proportion of patients remain on methotrexate therapy once started than is the case for other DMARDs. This reflects both efficacy and a relatively good tolerability profile. Methotrexate significantly suppresses inflammatory joint activity in a proportion of patients with established disease and early phase disease. It is also often effective in patients who have proved refractory to a number of other DMARDs. In addition to amelioration of symptoms and signs of disease, methotrexate inhibits the rate of progression of structural damage to joints, as assessed radiographically. This drug also has the advantage that the dose can be titrated according to therapeutic response, tolerability, and toxicity. A further advantage is that it is a useful combination partner that is widely used together with other DMARDs. Symptomatic benefits can be apparent after several weeks of therapy, but may take many months to reach a maximum level.

The therapeutic dose of methotrexate generally ranges from 7.5–25 mg on one day of the week only. The drug be taken by mouth, subcutaneous injection, or intramuscular injections. Use of parenteral methotrexate leads to serum concentrations of approximately 30% higher than achieved with oral methotrexate. As methotrexate depletes body stores of folate, folic acid supplements should be prescribed while patients are taking methotrexate. Typically, folic acid is given at a dose of 5 mg once weekly on the day after the methotrexate dose. Folic acid doses can be increased further; up to 5 mg daily if need be, particularly if the patient suffers from certain toxicities of methotrexate, including nausea and mouth ulceration.

Nausea is a relatively common side-effect of methotrexate therapy, and in more severe cases may result in vomiting or even anorexia. Other adverse events associated with this drug include hepatotoxicity and haemotological toxicity. The latter problem is reduced by regular folic acid supplementation and is less common if renal function is within the normal range. Pneumonitis is a rarer side effect of methotrexate and one that may resemble opportunist infections such as *Pneumocystis carinii* in immunosuppressed patients. Lymphoma has been reported as a rare association with methotrexate, although it should be remembered that there is an increased background rate of lymphoma in patients with active rheumatoid arthritis over that in the healthy population. One particular form of lymphoma associated with methotrexate may occur following Epstein-Barr virus infection, and this may resolve on withdrawal of methotrexate treatment. Expert histological typing is essential if lymphoma is suspected in order to ensure the most appropriate treatment.

Drug monitoring and minimising toxicities associated with methotrexate

Prior to commencing methotrexate, a baseline chest radiograph and biochemistry should be obtained. If any pulmonary complications that might represent a methotrexate pneumonitis occur, it is important to be able to compare the radiographic appearances with those of the baseline radiograph. Furthermore, significant baseline abnormality on the chest radiograph could be a relative contra-indication to use of methotrexate. Baseline urea, creatinine, and electrolytes give an indication of renal function. Methotrexate is best avoided in patients with renal insufficiency. Similarly, baseline biochemistry is an indication of any abnormalities in liver function test. It is also important to check baseline serology for hepatitis B or C exposure. Methotrexate should be used with caution, if at all, in patients with positive hepatitis B or C serology and also in those patients with transaminase levels raised

above 2.5 times the upper limit of the laboratory normal. In such circumstances, baseline liver biopsy is recommended and also in those patients where there are other risk factors for cirrhosis, such as significant alcohol intake.

Ideally, patients on methotrexate should avoid alcohol altogether or at least limit their consumption to modest levels in order to avoid hepatotoxic complications. Similarly, the combination of co-trimoxazol and methotrexate should be avoided, as this antibiotic decreases methotrexate excretion.

Methotrexate is contra-indicated in pregnancy because of potential risks of teratogenesis. For female patients of child-bearing age, appropriate education is important, and appropriate family planning must be emphasised. Methotrexate should be discontinued for at least one full menstrual cycle before attempting to conceive, but ideally for 3 months. Similarly, for male patients wishing to father children, methotrexate should be discontinued for up to 3 months and appropriate contraceptive methods used.

All patients on methotrexate should have regular blood monitoring tests, including a full blood count with platelets, liver function tests, and an acute phase marker such as an ESR. These tests should be undertaken every 4 weeks. If transaminase levels are elevated above 2.5 times the upper limit of normal, the methotrexate dose needs to be reduced or discontinued and the test repeated. If the test does not normalise, methotrexate will need to be discontinued. For the majority of patients, a simple dose adjustment is usually sufficient. It is always important to consider whether any other medication may be the cause of a raised transaminase and common culprits include NSAIDs such as diclofenac sodium.

Once patients are taking methotrexate, liver biopsy is not indicated unless liver function tests and, in particular, transaminase levels remain persistently elevated or albumin levels decrease.

Mechanism of action of methotrexate

Many biological effects of methotrexate have been described, although it is not fully understood which of these is the major mechanism of action, or indeed whether there are as-yet undescribed mechanisms. At the higher doses used in oncology treatments, methotrexate inhibits dihydrofolate reductase, which decreases levels of metabolically active reduced folates and, in turn, inhibits purine synthesis. However, it is unlikely that this mechanism is of major importance at the comparatively lower doses used in the treatment of rheumatoid arthritis. Methotrexate also inhibits the enzyme AICAR transformylase (5-aminoimidazole-4-carboxamide ribonucleotide). The consequence of this inhibition is to increase concentrations of the substrate AICAR, which in turn stimulates adenosine release. Adenosine has a number of potent anti-inflammatory properties and also inhibits neutrophil function.

Sulphasalazine

For many years, sulphasalazine was the most commonly used first-line DMARD in Europe, but it has now been superseded by methotrexate. The molecule comprises a sulphapyridine moiety and a 5-aminosalicylic acid moiety. It was originally generated in the belief that rheumatoid arthritis had an infectious aetiology and that an antibiotic component, coupled to an anti-inflammatory component, would be beneficial. Although sulphasalazine does have efficacy in rheumatoid arthritis and disease-modifying capability, its mode of action is uncertain.

The maintenance dosage of sulphasalazine is between 1–3 g/day in divided doses, though it is usually commenced at 500 mg once daily, and increased by 500 mg each week to the maintenance dose. More common side-effects of sulphasalazine include nausea, although this can be reduced by titrating the dose up gradually when commencing the drug, by use of enteric-coated tablets, and by taking the medication with food. Drug-related rashes can

occur, as can headache or dizziness. Neutropenia and liver enzyme abnormality can also be caused by sulphasalazine. Rarer toxicities include pulmonary infiltrates with eosinophilia. In men, oligospermia or even azoospermia is described; in the cases of couples having difficulty conceiving, if the male partner is taking sulphasalazine, this possibility needs to be considered, as it is reversible on withdrawal of the drug.

As in the case of methotrexate, sulphasalazine works well in combination with other DMARDs.

Patients on sulphasalazine should have routine blood monitoring tests. These comprise full blood count with platelets, creatinine, and liver function tests, taken at baseline and then once a month for the first 3 months of therapy and thereafter once every 3 months.

Hydroxychloroquine

Hydroxychloroquine is an anti-malarial and considered to be the least toxic of the DMARDs. It is rapidly absorbed, well tolerated, and effective in patients with the more mild disease expressions. It has beneficial effects on arthralgia and fatigue. It can be used in combination with other DMARDs. Hydroxychloroquine is the drug of choice among anti-malarials. Chloroquine is no longer recommended because of concerns regarding ocular toxicity. Hydroxychloroquine is used at a dose of 200–400 mg once daily. Symptomatic benefits take between 2–3 months to become apparent and patients should be warned of this. However, if there is no clinical benefit within 6 months, hydroxychloroquine should be considered ineffective in such a patient.

Side-effects include nausea, particularly early on in dosing, although this may lessen over time, particularly if the drug is started at half-dose and titrated upwards over 2–4 weeks. Less common side-effects include headache and dizziness, and myopathy may occur in high doses. Haemolysis is a rare complication that may arise in patients with glucose-6-phosphate dehydrogenase (G6PD) deficiency. A rash or skin hyperpigmentation may occur. The most important toxicity, however, is ocular, although this is extremely uncommon when hydroxychloroquine is used within the recommended dose range. Corneal deposits, extra-ocular muscular weakness, loss of accommodation, and a retinopathy may occur in about one of 40,000 patients. These changes are reversible if the drug is stopped rapidly but can lead to irreversible visual loss otherwise. Routine ophthalmological examination is no longer widely recommended but the patient should be cautioned that if there is any subjective change in colour vision that they should discontinue hydroxychloroquine straight away and seek specialist advice.

The mechanism of action of anti-malarials is not known. However, beneficial effects include an increase in lipoprotein (LDL) receptors, which helps to lower lipid levels. They also decrease insulin degradation, which has a protective effect against diabetes, and may also inhibit platelet aggregation and adhesion. They thus have cardioprotective effects.

Leflunomide

Leflunomide became available as a new DMARD agent for the treatment of rheumatoid arthritis in the late 1990s. In clinical trials, its efficacy was similar to that of methotrexate and sulphasalazine, in terms of improvement in symptoms and signs of disease. In addition, leflunomide retards the rate of radiographic progression to joints. Leflunomide represents an alternative DMARD choice for those patients who fail to respond to methotrexate or are unable to tolerate it. It can also be used in combination with methotrexate for patients demonstrating some improvement with methotrexate as a monotherapy, but nonetheless still have active disease.

The maintenance dose of leflunomide is between 10–20 mg once daily. To achieve a steady state, a loading dose of 100 mg daily for 3 days can be given; however, such a loading regimen may be associated with tolerability or

toxicity problems and, therefore, it is often preferable to use a starting dose of 20 mg once daily. The active metabolite of leflunomide has a half-life of 15 days. Both the parent compound and its active metabolite are extensively protein-bound and undergo further metabolism prior to excretion in the urine and faeces.

Evidence of symptomatic benefits may take 4–8 weeks to appear.

Side effects of leflunomide

Common side-effects include nausea and diarrhoea, the latter in over 15% of patients. This can lead to significant weight loss and there may also be associated vomiting. As with other DMARDs, skin rashes may occur and allergic reactions, particularly at the higher dose regimens. Alopecia may occur in over 5% of patients and this is reversible on drug cessation. Neutropenia is commoner than thrombocytopenia, both of which may be associated with leflunomide, and abnormalities in liver function tests may occur. Elevation of transaminase levels above 3 times the upper limit of normal is reported in between 2–4% of patients, with normalisation on cessation of the drug. Like methotrexate, leflunomide has a teratogenic potential and because of the persistence of active metabolite in tissues, particular care must be taken when using this drug for the treatment of women of child-bearing potential. Patients need to be educated about the possible risks to the fetus and cautioned to use adequate contraception. Similarly, males wishing to father a child will need to discontinue leflunomide prior to a planned conception. Because of the prolonged half-life of leflunomide and extremely long persistence in tissues, an enhanced drug elimination procedure has been developed for use prior to a planned pregnancy and also in the event of overdose or toxicity. It involves taking cholestyramine 8 g, three times daily for 11 days. Following cholestyramine treatment, women wishing to become pregnant should have blood tests taken on two occasions 14 days apart that document the active metabolite plasma level of leflunomide to be less than 0.02 µg/ml.

There have been reports of fatal hepatotoxicity due to leflunomide, the majority occurring within the first few months of initiating therapy and many in patients taking concomitant medications with potential for hepatotoxicity, such as methotrexate. For this reason, leflunomide should not be used in patients with hepatitis B or C and baseline serological testing should be undertaken before initiating the drug. Leflunomide should be used with caution when the patient is taking other potentially hepatotoxic drugs. As in the case of methotrexate, it is recommended that liver function tests are monitored on a monthly basis, particularly during the first 6 months of therapy. If the liver function tests become raised above 2 times the upper limit of normal or persistent minor elevations are noted, then the dose of leflunomide should be reduced until the patient is taking 10 mg once daily. If liver function tests become elevated greater than 3 times the upper limit of normal, then leflunomide should be stopped, and it may be necessary to consider use of a drug elimination protocol.

Mechanism of action of leflunomide

The active metabolite of leflunomide, A77 1726, is an inhibitor of dihydro-orotate dehydrogenase. This enzyme is responsible for the *de novo* synthesis of uridine; by decreasing its production, leflunomide treatment subsequently reduces pyrimidine biosynthesis. Because lymphocytes have low cellular pools of pyrimidine nucleotides, particularly in the case of B cells, they are sensitive to leflunomide. When cellular uridine is lowered below a critical level, there is activation of the tumour suppressor gene p53, and lymphocyte cell division becomes arrested in the G_1 stage of the cell cycle. Despite this, leflunomide treatment does not appear to be associated with an increased infection risk.

Gold salts

Until the early 1990s, intramuscular gold salts were the most frequently used DMARD agents. However, they have the disadvantage of a very slow onset of action and a high ratio of potentially serious toxicities to the numbers of patients responding to therapy. For this reason, gold preparations are much less frequently used now. However, in the small proportion of patients responding well to intramuscular gold, remissions can be achieved.

Intramuscular gold therapy is usually initiated with a test dose of 10 mg. In the absence of any undesirable reactions, further doses of between 25–50 mg are given once weekly until a significant response occurs or a total of 1 g has been administered. In the absence of any improvement by this time-point, therapy is usually discontinued on the grounds of lack of efficacy. On the other hand, if there is a significant improvement, the frequency of injection can be reduced to once every 2 weeks for several months; if remission is maintained, this can be reduced further to once every 3–4 weeks. The retention rate on gold is low, less than 10% of patients remaining on this therapy through 5 years of treatment, whether because of a lack of efficacy, toxicity, intolerance, or a combination of these. Oral gold was introduced as an alternative to the intramuscular preparation, but it has low efficacy, and also has frequent side effects, most notably involving the gastrointestinal tract, including diarrhoea.

Adverse events occur in over a third of patients on gold therapy. The most common side-effect is a rash that can vary from a simple pruritic erythematous patch to severe exfoliative dermatitis. Ulcerations and stomatitis can also occur and a mild mucocutaneous eruption is an indication to discontinue therapy temporarily. In the event of a resolution, treatment can be restarted at a lower dose of 10–15 mg weekly, titrating up to 50 mg weekly, with careful clinical monitoring. Up to 10% of patients have mild proteinuria, related to a gold-induced membranous glomerulonephropathy, but this can progress to the nephrotic range, and patients with proteinuria on dipstick testing should have a 24-hour urine collection for protein estimation. If proteinuria exceeds 500 mg in 24 hours, gold therapy should be stopped. Mild degrees of proteinuria generally resolve with cessation of treatment. Microscopic haematuria may also occur on gold therapy, but other causes must always be excluded. Less common but potentially serious side-effects include immune thrombocytopenia, granulocytopenia, and aplastic anaemia. These are all absolute indications to discontinue gold therapy. Intramuscular gold can also produce a nitritoid reaction, comprising flushing, dizziness, or fainting almost immediately after the injection.

As with the case of other DMARDs, careful monitoring can help to minimise serious problems. A full blood count, including platelet count and urine dip-sticking for proteinuria, should be undertaken prior to each gold injection.

The mechanism of action of gold salts is unknown, although several hypotheses have been postulated.

D-Penicillamine

As in the case of gold salts, D-penicillamine has been a widely used DMARD in previous years but is now rarely prescribed in the treatment of rheumatoid arthritis because of a number of potentially serious side-effects and because it takes 6 or more months for a significant clinical response to be seen, if at all. It used to be reserved for patients with persistent aggressive disease failing to achieve any significant improvement with less toxic agents. It may be useful in patients with extra-articular manifestations of rheumatoid arthritis, including vasculitis and Felty's syndrome.

It is administered as a once daily oral dose, starting on between 125–250 mg once daily, and titrating the dose upwards by 125–250 mg every 3 months to a maintenance dose of 750–1000 mg every day.

Side-effects include haematological disorders such as leukopenia and thrombocytopenia, membranous nephropathy, rashes, anorexia, nausea, and loss of taste. D-Penicillamine may also induce autoimmune syndromes such as myasthenia gravis, Goodpasture syndrome, drug-induced lupus, or pemphigus.

Monitoring requires monthly full blood counts with platelets and urinalysis for protein.

Drug treatment during pregnancy

Rheumatoid arthritis often improves during the course of pregnancy. This is likely to be due to the naturally occurring immunomodulatory effects taking place during the gravid state, including the release of endogenous steroids, with the purpose of preventing rejection of fetal tissue expressing paternal antigens foreign to the maternal immune system. Approximately three-quarters of women spontaneously remit during the course of pregnancy, and it is thus desirable to make use of this situation to minimise fetal exposure to potentially toxic medications. Despite this temporary improvement, relapse occurs in the majority within 6 months of delivery. Rheumatoid arthritis may present *de novo* during the postpartum period.

For those patients planning a family, it is important to discontinue therapies that might cause teratogenesis or otherwise harm the fetus. Withdrawal of methotrexate has been discussed above. However, it should also be remembered that it might take many months for the average couple to conceive, with the implication that disease may flare over this time period following withdrawal of methotrexate therapy and prior to conception. It is safe to use low-dose prednisolone throughout pregnancy without any risk to the fetus, and NSAIDs can be used in the first two trimesters. Sulphasalazine can be used with caution during pregnancy and is reported to be safe in patients with inflammatory bowel disease who continue to take the drug throughout their pregnancies. Folate supplementation is recommended in this circumstance. Methotrexate is contra-indicated in pregnancy and gold salts have been associated with congenital malformation. Hydroxychloroquine has been safely used in patients with lupus throughout the course of pregnancy, and similarly there is favourable experience in patients with rheumatoid arthritis. Azathioprine is also best avoided during pregnancy as various adverse effects have been described, including fetal retardation. D-Penicillamine and leflunomide should also be avoided. There is relatively little data available regarding biologicals targeting anti-TNF in the course of pregnancy, although emerging information suggests that etanercept can be used in patients with severe disease. Such treatment requires very careful monitoring.

All drugs must be used with caution in pregnancy. NSAIDs should be avoided in the third trimester because of the potential for premature closure of the ductus arteriosus, prolonged labour, and peripartum haemorrhage. If prednisolone use is deemed necessary during pregnancy, it is best to use the lowest dose that enables satisfactory symptom control. Potential complications of prednisolone therapy include worsening of maternal gestational diabetes, hypertension, and intra-uterine growth retardation.

Use of DMARDs during breast-feeding

Ibuprofen and naproxen can be used during breast-feeding but other NSAIDs should be avoided, in particular sulindac and indomethacin, because of enterohepatic circulation. Aspirin should be avoided in doses greater than 325 mg as the drug in breast milk may result in high plasma salicylate levels in the neonate. Corticosteroids are also excreted in the breast milk at a concentration of about 10–20% of the maternal dose. This means that there is a potential for growth retardation of the neonate during the breast-feeding period, particularly when the mother is taking prednisolone in a dose in excess of 20 mg

daily. Hydroxychloroquine is also secreted in breast milk and may potentially result in infant's retinal toxicity. Sulphasalazine can be used during lactation but it is considered best to avoid methotrexate during this period, although there is little excretion in breast milk.

In practice, for those women wishing to breast-feed whose disease flares early in the postpartum period, it may be best to advise them to breast-feed for a short time only and then to substitute bottle feeding and recommence a suitable drug regimen to suppress their synovitis effectively.

Combination non-biological DMARD therapy

Over the last 20 years or more, there have been a number of attempts to improve the outcomes achievable with non-biological DMARD therapies. In particular, there has been wide-spread acceptance of the excellent efficacy associated with methotrexate therapy, most marked when there is a rapid dose titration to between 20–25 mg once weekly, if tolerated. It has also become common-place to use two or more DMARDs concomitantly in the belief that there are added benefits in terms of efficacy with surprisingly little increase in toxicity or tolerability problems. Although the major mechanisms of action of many of the most widely used DMARDs are not well defined, the rationale for combination therapy is to target a number of distinct inflammatory pathways involved in the pathogenesis of inflammatory joint disease, and thus to suppress synovitis and accompanying tissue destruction more completely. Although the use of combination strategies has become very popular, the clinical trial data for these approaches is not always easy to interpret and there is surprisingly little unequivocal evidence to support the superiority of combination regimens with non-biological DMARD therapies.[9] This is in part because many of the clinical trials of combination therapy allow differences in the use of corticosteroids in the treatment arms.

A number of approaches have been used in the investigation of strategies for combination DMARD therapies. These approaches, which are also used in clinical practice, include: (i) a parallel strategy in which DMARDs are initiated simultaneously; (ii) step-up combination strategy, in which one DMARD is added to the background of another DMARD, to which there may have been a partial response; and (iii) a step-down strategy, in which combination DMARDs are initiated simultaneously with subsequent sequential withdrawal, following the attainment of a pre-set clinical benefit.

The design of clinical trials of combination DMARD therapy published up until the mid-1990s followed a parallel strategy, in which the combination therapy is compared with monotherapy. It is important to remember that the demonstration of superior efficacy in the combination therapy arm does not necessarily imply that the combination has an additive benefit. It may be that one of the combination drugs is in fact significantly more efficacious than the monotherapy comparator. An example would be the demonstration that the combination of methotrexate and hydroxychloroquine is more effective than hydroxychloroquine as a monotherapy.[10] In comparison, the finding that combined treatment with methotrexate and hydroxychloroquine has a better outcome than treatment with methotrexate alone is a more clinically meaningful finding.[11] Even so, there was only a marginal increase in benefit for the methotrexate and hydroxychloroquine combination over that of methotrexate alone, and less toxicity in the monotherapy group.

Interpretation of the findings of many parallel strategy trials is made more difficult by the absence of treatment group blinding. One particularly important open-label, parallel group, randomised trial was conducted in Finland – the so-called Fin-RACo study.[12] This 2-year, multicentre study investigated the efficacy and tolerability of combination therapy with sulphasalazine, methotrexate, hydroxychloroquine and prednisolone, compared

with a single DMARD with or without prednisolone in the treatment of early rheumatoid arthritis. a total of 199 patients were randomised and 195 of these started treatment. All 98 patients assigned to the single DMARD arm were started on sulphasalazine; in 51 of these patients, methotrexate was later substituted. Corticosteroid use was mandatory in the combination arm but not required in the monotherapy arm, in which only 27% of patients received corticosteroids from the start of therapy. Delayed initiation of corticosteroids was allowed up to 93 weeks from baseline in the DMARD monotherapy group. These differences in corticosteroid usage between the two study groups create some difficulties in interpretation of the findings. The remission frequencies were significantly higher in the combination arm at both 1 and 2 years. Radiographic progression was also less in the combination arm (Fig. 6.4). However, ACR responses were not statistically different. Interestingly, in the monotherapy arm, a short delay in treatment of greater than 4 months after diagnosis significantly reduced the remission rate at 2 years (Fig. 6.5). The combination therapy was not associated with more adverse events than the single DMARD treatment. These findings have been widely used to support the use of early combination therapy but do not exclude the possibility that the differences in the two groups could be accounted for on the basis of mandatory early steroid treatment.

Another important parallel strategy study that has been widely reported to demonstrate the superior efficacy of the triple DMARD combination, comprising methotrexate, hydroxychloroquine, and sulphasalazine, is that by O'Dell and colleagues in established rheumatoid arthritis, and had the benefit of a double-blind, randomised design. Of the triple DMARD combination group, 77% achieved a 50% improvement at 9 months, and maintained at least that degree of improvement for 2 years without evidence of major drug toxicity. This contrasted with 33%

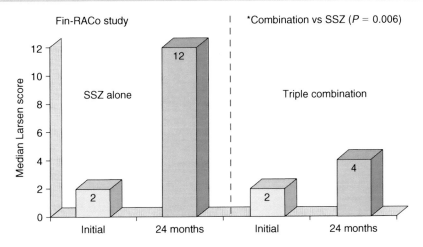

Figure 6.4
Radiographic outcomes in FinCO-RA study of combination therapy in early rheumatoid arthritis. Based on data from Möttönen et al.[12] Reprinted with permission of Wiley–Liss, Inc., a subsidiary of John Wiley & Sons, Inc., © 2002, John Wiley & Sons.

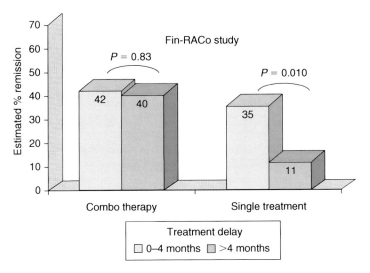

Figure 6.5
Short delay of therapy predicts remission at 2 years for patients on monotherapy. Based on data from Möttönen et al.[12] Reprinted with permission of Wiley–Liss, Inc., a subsidiary of John Wiley & Sons, Inc., © 2002, John Wiley & Sons.

of patients receiving methotrexate therapy alone and 40% of patients treated with sulphasalazine and hydroxychloroquine.[13] However, in the latter treatment group, sulphasalazine was given at the low dose of 1 g daily. Radiographic progression was not reported in this study.

There is data to suggest a biological mechanism whereby sulphasalazine might diminish the efficacy of methotrexate.[14] At clinically relevant plasma concentrations, sulphasalazine interacts with reduced folate carrier, the dominant cell membrane transporter for natural folates and methotrexate. These findings argue in favour of the use of folate supplementation during sulphasalazine treatment in the same way as is used during methotrexate therapy. These observations may also explain the paucity of clinical trial data unequivocally supporting superiority of the combination of methotrexate and sulphasalazine over either of the components.[15,16] However, there are radiographic data from open-label parallel strategy trials where assessors blinded to the clinical outcome evaluated radiographs. For example, in established rheumatoid arthritis, the triple DMARD therapy combination of methotrexate, hydroxychloroquine, and sulphasalazine, as well as the dual DMARD therapy combinations of either methotrexate and hydroxychloroquine or methotrexate and sulphasalazine, gave superior radiographic or clinical outcomes to patients in the monotherapy group in which patients received a single DMARD comprising either methotrexate, sulphasalazine, or hydroxychloroquine. Again, however, the interpretation of radiographic superiority of the combination group is open to question because a third of those patients in the monotherapy group, namely, those on hydroxychloroquine alone, would not be anticipated to gain much by way of protection against structural damage; therefore, the chosen analyses bias in favour of the combination therapy groups, which include either methotrexate or sulphasalazine, both of which are known to have a more marked disease-modifying effect than hydroxychloroquine.

Step-up clinical trial strategies

From the mid-1990s onwards, the step-up strategy design has predominated in clinical trials of pharmacotherapeutics for rheumatoid arthritis. An important example was an investigation of the effects of addition of cyclosporin A to patients with active, established rheumatoid arthritis despite pre-existing methotrexate therapy. This was compared with the addition of placebo to patients on existing methotrexate therapy.[17] In this study, 48% of patients in the step-up

combination therapy group achieved ACR 20% responses as compared with 16% of patients in the methotrexate monotherapy group. However, it is not clear from this study whether the higher proportion of responders in the methotrexate and cyclosporin arm is due to an additive effect of the combination or due to the cyclosporin alone. That the latter might be the case would be supported by the findings of a double-blind, randomised controlled parallel group study comparing cyclosporin and methotrexate with cyclosporin and placebo.[18] In this study, 47% of patients treated with cyclosporin and placebo achieved an ACR 20% response. This figure is in line with the percentage of responders in the combination therapy arm in the Tugwell et al. study,[17] although it is always important to be cautious in comparing response findings in this way across patient populations in different clinical trials. Gerards et al.[18] reported a significantly higher proportion of responders among the cyclosporin and methotrexate combination group at the ACR 50 level (48% versus 25% of patients in the cyclosporin and placebo group). Similarly, while these data have been interpreted as favouring combination DMARD therapy, because there was no methotrexate and placebo arm in this study, it cannot be said unequivocally that the findings in this combination arm could not be accounted for on the basis of a methotrexate effect rather than an additive effect.

Another DMARD combination that has had limited popularity is that of leflunomide together with methotrexate, largely because of the increased toxicity observed when the drugs are taken together.[19] As with other previously discussed papers, it is not entirely clear whether the superior ACR responses at the 20%, 50%, and 70% level observed when leflunomide is added to patients on a stable dose of methotrexate as compared to addition of placebo really reflects an additive benefit or simply a superior efficacy with leflunomide in this particular patient population. That this may indeed be the case is suggested by other studies comparing leflunomide as a monotherapy with other DMARD monotherapies such as sulphasalazine[20] or methotrexate.[21,22] Although the patient populations in these studies are not strictly comparable, the reported ACR response rates in the leflunomide arms are at least as good as that reported for the methotrexate and leflunomide combination in the study by Kremer et al.[19] These observations cast some doubt on the contention that the combination of methotrexate and leflunomide is superior to that of leflunomide alone, although it does suggest that in this population of patients with active disease despite methotrexate, that further improvement could be gained by addition of leflunomide. Another study compared the efficacy and safety of adding sulphasalazine to leflunomide treatment with switching to sulphasalazine alone in rheumatoid patients with an inadequate response to leflunomide as a monotherapy.[23] Although the patient numbers were small, there was no demonstrable benefit in combining leflunomide with sulphasalazine compared with switching to sulphasalazine alone in patients responding inadequately to leflunomide. Furthermore, there was more toxicity associated with the combination.

Sequential step-up combination DMARD therapy has become a popular approach to treatment of patients with active rheumatoid arthritis, and is often employed prior to the introduction of biological therapies. However, there are very few studies to date confirming the clinical impression that addition of hydroxychloroquine, sulphasalazine, or both is effective in patients with active disease who have only achieved a partial therapeutic response on maximally tolerated methotrexate doses. This is an important question because, despite the popularity of methotrexate as a first-line DMARD, the majority of patients will not achieve a 50% improvement with this drug as a monotherapy. A small, open-label, controlled trial investigating this issue reported a substantial improvement when both sulphasalazine and hydroxychloroquine were added to methotrexate partial responders, with a lower magnitude of improvement when either

hydroxychloroquine or sulphasalazine alone were added to pre-existing methotrexate therapy.[24]

Step-down combination DMARD strategies

The step-down strategy is perhaps best exemplified by the COBRA trial (COmbinatietherapie Bij Reumatoide Artritis). This trial evaluated step-down combination therapy with prednisolone, methotrexate, and sulphasalazine versus sulphasalazine as a monotherapy.[25] The primary outcomes measured were disease activity, radiological damage, and functional ability. The low-dose methotrexate and sulphasalazine in combination with high-dose corticosteroid had superior efficacy to sulphasalazine alone in terms of reduction in joint damage despite similar reductions in symptoms and signs at the 1-year end-point after steroid withdrawal. This finding may be a reflection of the more rapid suppression of symptoms and signs in the combination therapy group, resulting in a significantly lower mean time-averaged DAS 28, despite the convergence of the two treatment strategies in terms of inflammatory load at the end of 1 year. During a 4–5 year follow-up period, the radiographic progression was slower in the group originally treated with combination therapy compared with the sulphasalazine monotherapy group, with a Sharp score progression rate of 8.6 points per year in the monotherapy group versus 5.6 in the COBRA group.[26] Thus an initial 6-month cycle of intensive combination treatment that included high-dose corticosteroids resulted in sustained suppression of the rate of radiographic progression in patients with early rheumatoid arthritis independently of their subsequent anti-rheumatic therapy.

In clinical practice, corticosteroids have widely been used in step-down strategies as a bridging therapy because of their rapid suppression of symptoms and signs of disease, while allowing time for a more slowly acting DMARD to take effect. In a study of 59 patients commencing intramuscular gold therapy, patients were randomised to receive three doses of 120 mg intramuscular depomethylprednisolone, or a matching placebo at weeks 0, 4, and 8, in addition to their gold treatment. Those receiving corticosteroid had a more rapid improvement in disease activity but this initial advantage, evident for the first 12 weeks, was lost by 24 weeks.[27] Similar short-term benefits of corticosteroids used as a bridging therapy have been reported with oral prednisolone. Forty patients receiving gold therapy were randomised to receive either prednisolone or placebo treatment for 18 weeks. Prednisolone was given at 10 mg daily for the first 12 weeks then 7.5 mg daily for weeks 13 and 14, 5 mg daily for weeks 15 and 16, and 2.5 mg daily in weeks 17 and 18. Disease activity was significantly lower in the group receiving corticosteroids as early as week 1, and this benefit continued up to week 12. However, a rebound deterioration was noticed at weeks 20 and 24 in over half of the responders.[28]

More recently, in a multicentre Dutch study comparing four different treatment strategies in the early phase of rheumatoid arthritis, initial use of the COBRA regimen step-down approach showed superiority with regard to remission rates and radiographic progression over a sequential monotherapy and step-up combination therapy strategy. Interestingly, radiographic progression was very similar in the groups assigned to sequential monotherapy and step-up combination therapy. Certainly, there was not compelling evidence to suggest superiority of a step-up combination strategy over sequential switching of DMARDs and the findings would be consistent with the hypothesis that much of the apparent benefit of the early combination therapy intervention was attributable to high-dose corticosteroids.[29] However, it should be noted that high-dose steroids as used in the COBRA regimen, which begins with prednisolone at 60 mg daily, is disliked by patients, and there are always concerns about corticosteroid toxicities. For this reason, very few rheumatologists use the COBRA regimen as originally described, although there is much to be said in support of

a modified regimen starting at lower prednisolone doses with subsequent taper.

Summary

The range of therapies in the pharmacological armamentarium for rheumatoid arthritis fall into one of four broad categories – NSAIDs, corticosteroids, DMARDs and biological agents. NSAIDs and corticosteroids have a useful place in the control of symptoms and signs of rheumatoid arthritis. DMARDs and biological therapies also help to suppress synovitis and to retard its destructive sequelae. Judicious use of the available agents, tailored to individual needs, allows optimum symptom control and the most favourable long-term outcomes. For the majority of patients presenting with rheumatoid arthritis in the present era, there is every reason to paint an optimistic picture regarding future health prospects.

References

1. Burke TA, Goldstein JL, Pettit AD, Maurath CJ, Zhao SZ, Zabinski RA. Increased upper gastrointestinal (UGI) distress among arthritis patients treated with NSAIDs as compared to celecoxib and placebo. *Value Health* 1999; **2**: 154–5.

2. Graham DY, Smith JL. Gastroduodenal complications of chronic NSAID therapy. *Am J Gastroenterol* 1988; **83**: 1081–4.

3. Blower AL, Brooks A, Fenn GC et al. Emergency admissions for upper gastrointestinal disease and their relation to NSAID use. *Aliment Pharmacol Ther* 1997; **11**: 283–91.

4. Singh G, Ramey DR, Morfeld D, Shi H, Hatoum HT, Fries JF. Gastrointestinal tract complications of nonsteroidal anti-inflammatory drug treatment in rheumatoid arthritis. A prospective observational cohort study. *Arch Intern Med* 1996; **156**: 1530–6.

5. Bombardier C, Laine L, Reicin A et al. and VIGOR Study Group. Comparison of upper gastrointestinal toxicity of rofecoxib and naproxen in patients with rheumatoid arthritis. *N Engl J Med* 2000; **343**: 1520–8.

6. Silverstein FE, Faich G, Goldstein JL et al. Gastrointestinal toxicity with celecoxib vs nonsteroidal anti-inflammatory drugs for osteoarthritis and rheumatoid arthritis: the CLASS study: a randomized controlled trial. Celecoxib Long-term Arthritis Safety Study. *JAMA* 2000; **284**: 1247–55.

7. Bresalier RS, Sandler RS, Quan H et al. and Adenomatous Polyp Prevention on Vioxx (APPROVe) Trial Investigators.

Cardiovascular events associated with rofecoxib in a colorectal adenoma chemoprevention trial. *N Engl J Med* 2005; **352**: 1092–102.

8. Nussmeier NA, Whelton AA, Brown MT *et al.* Complications of the COX-2 inhibitors parecoxib and valdecoxib after cardiac surgery. *N Engl J Med* 2005; **352**: 1081–91.

9. Smolen JS, Aletaha D, Keystone E. Superior efficacy of combination therapy for rheumatoid arthritis: fact or fiction? *Arthritis Rheum* 2005; **52**: 2975–83.

10. Trnavsky K, Gatterova J, Linduskova M, Peliskova Z. Combination therapy with hydroxychloroquine and methotrexate in rheumatoid arthritis. *Z Rheumatol* 1993; **52**: 292–6.

11. Ferraz MB, Pinheiro GR, Helfenstein M *et al.* Combination therapy with methotrexate and chloroquine in rheumatoid arthritis. A multicenter randomized placebo-controlled trial. *Scand J Rheumatol* 1994; **23**: 231–6.

12. Möttönen T, Hannonen P, Korpela M, *et al.* Delay to institution of therapy and induction of remission using single-drug or combination-disease-modifying antirheumatic drug therapy in early rheumatoid arthritis. *Arthritis Rheum* 2002; **46**: 894–8.

13. O'Dell JR, Haire CE, Erikson N *et al.* Treatment of rheumatoid arthritis with methotrexate alone, sulfasalazine and hydroxychloroquine, or a combination of all three medications. *N Engl J Med* 1996; **334**: 1287–91.

14. Jansen G, van der Heijden J, Oerlemans R *et al.* Sulfasalazine is a potent inhibitor of the reduced folate carrier: implications for combination therapies with methotrexate in rheumatoid arthritis. *Arthritis Rheum* 2004; **50**: 2130–9.

15. Dougados M, Combe B, Cantagrel A *et al.* Combination therapy in early rheumatoid arthritis: a randomised, controlled, double blind 52 week clinical trial of sulphasalazine and methotrexate compared with the single components. *Ann Rheum Dis* 1999; **58**: 220–5.

16. Haagsma CJ, van Riel PL, de Jong AJ, van de Putte LB. Combination of sulphasalazine and methotrexate versus the single components in early rheumatoid arthritis: a randomized, controlled, double-blind, 52 week clinical trial. *Br J Rheumatol* 1997; **36**: 1082–8.

17. Tugwell P, Pincus T, Yocum D *et al.* Combination therapy with cyclosporine and methotrexate in severe rheumatoid arthritis. The Methotrexate-Cyclosporine Combination Study Group. *N Engl J Med* 1995; **333**: 137–41.

18. Gerards AH, Landewe RB, Prins AP *et al.* Cyclosporin A monotherapy versus cyclosporin A and methotrexate combination therapy in patients with early rheumatoid arthritis: a double blind randomised placebo controlled trial. *Ann Rheum Dis* 2003; **62**: 291–6.

19. Kremer JM, Genovese MC, Cannon GW *et al.* Concomitant leflunomide therapy in patients with active rheumatoid arthritis despite stable doses of methotrexate. A randomized, double-blind, placebo-controlled trial. *Ann Intern Med* 2002; **137**: 726–33.

20. Smolen JS, Kalden JR, Scott DL *et al.* Efficacy and safety of leflunomide compared with placebo and sulphasalazine in active rheumatoid arthritis: a double-blind, randomised, multicentre trial. European Leflunomide Study Group. *Lancet* 1999; **353**: 259–66.

21. Strand V, Cohen S, Schiff M *et al.* Treatment of active rheumatoid arthritis with leflunomide compared with placebo and methotrexate. Leflunomide Rheumatoid Arthritis Investigators Group. *Arch Intern Med* 1999; **159**: 2542–50.

22. Emery P, Breedveld FC, Lemmel EM *et al.* A comparison of the efficacy and safety of leflunomide and methotrexate for the treatment of rheumatoid arthritis. *Rheumatology (Oxford)* 2000; **39**: 655–65.

23. Klareskog L, Gaubitz M, Rodriguez-Valverde V, Malaise M, Dougados M, Wajdula J. A long-term, open-label trial of the safety and efficacy of etanercept (ENBREL(R)) in patients with rheumatoid arthritis not treated with other DMARDs (3-year interim report). *Ann Rheum Dis* 2006; doi:10.1136/ard.2005.038349.

24. O'Dell J. Conventional DMARD options for patients with a suboptimal response to methotrexate. *J Rheumatol Suppl* 2001; **62**: 21–6.

25. Boers M, Verhoeven AC, Markusse HM *et al.* Randomised comparison of combined step-down prednisolone, methotrexate and sulphasalazine with sulphasalazine alone in early rheumatoid arthritis. *Lancet* 1997; **350**: 309–18.

26. Landewe RB, Boers M, Verhoeven AC *et al.* COBRA combination therapy in patients with early rheumatoid arthritis: long-term structural benefits of a brief intervention. *Arthritis Rheum* 2002; **46**: 347–56.

27. Corkill MM, Kirkham BW, Chikanza IC, Gibson T, Panayi GS. Intramuscular depot methylprednisolone induction of chrysotherapy in rheumatoid arthritis: a 24-week randomized controlled trial. *Br J Rheumatol* 1990; **29**: 274–9.

28. van Gestel AM, Laan RF, Haagsma CJ, van de Putte LB, van Riel PL. Oral steroids as bridge therapy in rheumatoid arthritis patients starting with parenteral gold. A randomized double-blind placebo-controlled trial. *Br J Rheumatol* 1995; **34**: 347–51.

29. Goekoop-Ruiterman YP, de Vries-Bouwstra JK, Allaart CF *et al.* Clinical and radiographic outcomes of four different treatment strategies in patients with early rheumatoid arthritis (the BeSt study): a randomized, controlled trial. *Arthritis Rheum* 2005; **52**: 3381–90.

7 Biological therapies for rheumatoid arthritis targeting TNF-α and IL-1

What is a biological therapy?
Biological therapies targeting TNF-α
Biological therapies targeting IL-1
Combination anti-cytokine therapies
Conclusions

What is a biological therapy?

So-called 'biologics' are protein-based drugs derived from living organisms that are designed either to inhibit or augment a specific component of the immune system. Examples include antibodies directed against very specific molecular components of the immune response, for example, pro-inflammatory cytokines, or naturally occurring cytokine inhibitors such as IL-1 receptor antagonist (IL-1ra). A potential advantage of a highly targeted therapeutic is the avoidance of toxic effects that a drug may have on molecular pathways other than their effects on the primary therapeutic target. Even so, where a biological targets a single component of the immune system, mechanism-related toxicity may still arise.

The primary cause of rheumatoid arthritis remains unknown. Nonetheless, advances in molecular technology have facilitated identification of numerous novel therapeutic targets, including cytokines, cell subsets, and other molecules, such as those involved in signalling pathways, that contribute to the inflammatory and destructive components of rheumatoid arthritis. Concurrent advances in biotechnology made it possible to produce abundant, high-quality, chimerised mouse–human or even completely human monoclonal antibodies with specificity for relevant disease molecules. Other approaches to blocking pro-inflammatory molecules include the use of naturally occurring soluble receptors or inhibitory proteins.

Biological therapies targeting TNF-α

At the present time, biologicals represent the only available class of specific TNF inhibitors available for clinical practice. Three drugs are currently approved (Fig. 7.1): (i) infliximab (Remicade), a chimeric monoclonal anti-TNF-α antibody comprising a human IgG-1κ antibody with a mouse SV fragment of high affinity and neutralising capacity; (ii) adalimumab (Humira), a monoclonal human antibody produced by phage display; and (iii) etanercept (Enbrel), an engineered p75 TNF receptor dimer with a fully human amino acid sequence linked to the Fc portion of human IgG_1. The monoclonal antibodies have specificity for TNF-α. Binding assays using radioactively labelled TNF-α demonstrate that antibodies such as infliximab bind both monomeric (inactive) and trimeric (biologically active) forms of soluble TNF-α.[1] In contrast, the fusion protein etanercept acts as a competitive inhibitor of TNF-α and can also bind lympotoxin (TNF-β). Etanercept forms relatively unstable complexes with TNF-α, allowing dissociation and the potential to form a reservoir for binding TNF-α.[1] Aside from the three currently approved biological TNF inhibitors for rheumatoid arthritis, others are in development, including certolizumab pegol, (formerly known as CDP-870, now Cimzia), a pegylated Fab fragment which can be produced in *Escherichia coli*.[2]

Rationale for TNF blockade in the treatment of rheumatoid arthritis

The predicted clinical success of anti-TNF therapy was based on four lines of evidence:

- the demonstration of rheumatoid arthritis synovial tissue expression of TNF-α and its receptors[3]

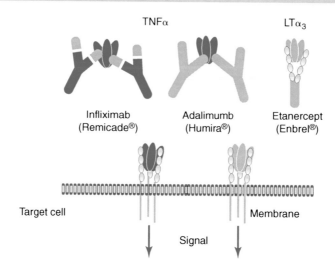

Figure 7.1
There are three currently licensed biological inhibitors of TNF-α for the treatment of rheumatoid arthritis. Infliximab is a chimeric monoclonal antibody that includes murine amino-acid sequences in the variable region of the immunoglobulin. Adalimumab is a monoclonal antibody with a fully human amino-acid sequence and etanercept is a fusion protein comprising an engineered p75 TNF receptor dimer with a fully human amino-acid sequence linked to the Fc portion of human IgG_1.

- evidence from *in vitro* experiments employing dissociated synovial cell cultures pointing to TNF-α as a regulator of many other pro-inflammatory cytokines[4-6]

- a number of independent *in vivo* studies demonstrating that blockade of bioactive TNF in murine collagen-induced arthritis could ameliorate clinical symptoms and prevent joint destruction in established disease[7]

- in a murine model, the over-expression of a human TNF-α transgene modified at its 3'-end to prevent degradation of its mRNA was associated with the development of a destructive form of polyarthritis 4–6 weeks after birth. This could be prevented by administration of a monoclonal antibody with specificity for human TNF.[8]

Tissue expression of an extensive range of pro-inflammatory cytokines in human synovial samples, regardless of differences in donor disease duration, severity, or even drug therapy, has been confirmed in studies from a number of laboratories. These findings imply that there is prolonged expression of cytokines in the rheumatoid joint, contrasting with the transient production induced by mitogenic stimulation. This hypothesis was confirmed following the observation that pro-inflammatory cytokines are produced over several days in dissociated rheumatoid arthritis synovial membrane cell cultures in the absence of extrinsic stimulation.[9] This finding suggested that one or more soluble factors regulating prolonged cytokine synthesis were present within the rheumatoid arthritis synovial membrane cultures. These cultures comprise a heterogeneous population of cells producing numerous cytokine and other non-cytokine molecular messengers. A key observation to emerge using this cell culture system was that addition of anti-TNF antibodies strikingly reduced the production of other pro-inflammatory cytokines including IL-1, GM-CSF, IL-6, and IL-8.[4] Furthermore, using the same rheumatoid arthritis synovial cell culture system, blockade of IL-1 by means of the IL-1 receptor antagonists results in reduced IL-6 and IL-8 production but not that of TNF-α.[5] These observations led to the formulation of the hypothesis that TNF-α occupies a dominant position at the apex of a pro-inflammatory cytokine network. At the time of these experimental findings, in the early 1990s, TNF-α had also been described as a pleiotropic cytokine with biological properties that included enhanced synovial proliferation, production of prostaglandins and metalloproteinases,[10] as well as regulation of other pro-inflammatory cytokines. For all these reasons, TNF-α was considered to represent a potential therapeutic target in rheumatoid arthritis.

The first data *in vivo* to support the hypothesis that TNF-α is a good therapeutic target for inflammatory arthritis came from studies of murine collagen-induced arthritis. Monoclonal anti-TNF antibodies or soluble TNF receptor-Fc fusion proteins, administered either during the induction phase of arthritis or, more importantly, in the established phase of disease after the onset of symptoms, were able to ameliorate clinical features and significantly inhibit joint destruction.[11,12] Further unequivocal validation of TNF-α as a therapeutic target came following the administration of biological agents to patients with rheumatoid arthritis.

Clinical studies of anti-TNF therapy

Learning point

Clinical benefits

- reduction of symptoms, including pain, stiffness, and lethargy

- reduction in signs of active disease, including joint swelling and tenderness

- reduction in cartilage and bone damage

- remission induction

- preservation and improvement of functional status

Data from numerous clinical trials with the anti-TNF agents infliximab, etanercept, and adalimumab have confirmed the validity of TNF-α as a therapeutic target in rheumatoid arthritis. Proof of principle for TNF-α blockade was initially established in an open-label study in which infliximab was administered intravenously in divided doses over 2 weeks (either 10 mg/kg a fortnight apart, or four doses of 5 mg/kg every 4 days). The results clearly demonstrated that these relatively large doses of antibody were tolerated without any immediate adverse reaction.[13] Although these early studies were not primarily designed to test efficacy, a remarkable reduction in pain, stiffness, swelling, and joint tenderness was observed within 24 hours, with maximum benefit at around 2–4 weeks, and sustained for the entire 8-week duration of the study in the majority of patients. Relief of fatigue within hours of the infusion was consistently reported. Subsequent studies in both the early and established phases of disease confirm that long-term, repeated use of anti-TNF agents results in sustained improvement in symptoms and signs of disease in the majority of patients.[14–23]

In studies of rheumatoid populations having failed to respond adequately after exposure to multiple DMARD therapies, with active disease despite on-going methotrexate therapy, between 50–70% of patients are reported to achieve an ACR 20 response level at 6 months, as compared to between 20–30% of patients treated with methotrexate alone.[24–26]

However, it is important to note that caution should be applied when comparing differences between proportions of responders or magnitude of response between studies, as the nature of the study populations are very different with respect to baseline disease activity and rate of structural damage to joints. At the more stringent 50% ACR response level, the difference between the proportion of patients with established disease responding on methotrexate alone and those responding on the combination of methotrexate and a TNF inhibitor is approximately 20–40% at 1 year and similarly, at the ACR 70% response level, about 15% of the study population.[24-26]

It is of note that most TNF inhibitors have been evaluated using a step-up design in patients with active disease despite methotrexate therapy, who then received either the TNF inhibitor or placebo. In many of these trials, however, a biological monotherapy arm was absent. Nonetheless, in a study of patients with an inadequate response to methotrexate, infliximab was administered at a dose of 1, 3, or 10 mg/kg, with or without a fixed low dose of methotrexate, while control groups were treated with placebo infusions and methotrexate.[27] In this trial, the duration of response to repeated biological administration was inversely related to the production of human anti-chimeric antibodies to the infliximab. Higher doses of infliximab were found to be less immunogenic than a low dose of 1 mg/kg, and concomitant methotrexate administration further reduced the occurrence of human anti-chimeric antibody responses. Although reduced immunogenicity of the biological agent administered may be one mechanism whereby methotrexate has an additive or synergistic benefit when used in combination with TNF inhibitors, it is likely that there are other effects beyond this mediated through complementary mechanism of action, although these have yet to be fully elucidated.

In the TEMPO study (Trial of Etanercept and Methotrexate with radiographic Patient Outcomes), the combination of methotrexate with etanercept was clearly superior to that of either methotrexate or etanercept alone.[17] Similarly, in the PREMIER study (a prospective, multicentre, randomised, double-blind, active comparator-controlled, parallel groups study comparing the fully human monoclonal anti-TNF antibody D2E7 given every second week with methotrexate given weekly, and the combination of D2E7 and methotrexate administered over 2 years in patients with early rheumatoid arthritis), the combination of

adalimumab and methotrexate consistently demonstrated superior efficacy in every area over either methotrexate or adalimumab as monotherapies.[21] In this study at week 52, 43% of patients on combination therapy achieved remission by DAS 28 criteria of less than 2.6 as compared with 23% of patients receiving adalimumab alone and 21% of patients receiving methotrexate alone. In the ASPIRE study of infliximab in early rheumatoid arthritis, 17% of patients receiving 6 mg/kg of infliximab together with methotrexate achieved an ACR 70 response for 6 or more consecutive months and 12% of patients receiving infliximab at 3 mg/kg together with methotrexate. This contrasted with under 8% of patients on methotrexate alone.[18] Of patients on methotrexate alone, 15% achieved remission criteria by DAS 28 at week 54, whereas the addition of infliximab at 3 mg/kg enhanced this figure to 21%, and further to 31% at a dose of 6 mg/kg.

One of the early studies to look at biomarkers after anti-TNF therapy demonstrated dose-dependent reductions in serum concentrations of pro-matrix metalloproteinase 1 and pro-matrix metalloproteinase 3.[28] These reductions in mediators of cartilage degradation predicted that TNF blockade might have the benefit of significant inhibition of radiographic damage to joints. That this was indeed the case was confirmed in the 54-week analyses from the ATTRACT study.[16] In this trial, infliximab, at doses of 3 mg/kg or 10 mg/kg, given every 4 or 8 weeks, when added to therapeutic doses of methotrexate was found to give sustained reduction in symptoms and signs of disease that were significantly greater than the reduction associated with methotrexate alone. In patients treated with methotrexate as a monotherapy, joint space narrowing and erosions progressed as anticipated. In contrast, therapy with infliximab plus methotrexate prevented the progressive joint damage characteristic of rheumatoid arthritis and even resulted in improvement in the radiographic score from baseline in a significant percentage of patients.[16]

Combination therapy halted progression of joint damage not only with limited radiographic destruction at baseline, but also in those with extensive damage. Similar findings have been reported for etanercept. When administered together with methotrexate, the combination was significantly better in inhibition of radiographic progression compared with methotrexate or etanercept alone, in a population of patients who were methotrexate-naive at study entry.[17] Very similar findings have been reported for adalimumab given in combination with methotrexate in the established phase of disease.[26]

There is also good evidence that antibodies targeting TNF significantly inhibit progression of structural damage in the early phase of disease.[18,21] These observations confirm the pathogenic role of TNF-α in the early phase of rheumatoid arthritis and suggest that, in the proportion of patients with high likelihood of radiographic progression, early intervention with a TNF inhibitor together with methotrexate may provide long-term benefits in terms of functional capability by preserving joint integrity.[19] Surprisingly, significant inhibition of radiographic damage has even been reported in those patients failing to achieve a clinical response at the ACR 20 level.[29] This fascinating observation in effect defines a subpopulation in whom there is a dissociation between inflammatory and destructive pathways.

Changes in functional status are assessed by means of the HAQ score. It has been determined that an improvement from baseline of 0.25 in HAQ score represents a clinically meaningful change. There is data for all three currently available anti-TNF inhibitors to show that repeated therapy over time, in particular when an anti-TNF agent is combined with methotrexate, leads to significant improvement in physical function and quality of life.[17,26,30]

Preservation or improvement of function is a particularly important goal of therapy in the early phases of disease. In the ASPIRE study, 60% of patients treated with methotrexate as a monotherapy achieved an improvement in HAQ exceeding 0.3, whereas 71% of all patients receiving infliximab together with methotrexate achieved an improvement of this magnitude.[18] Similarly, in the PREMIER study, patients receiving adalimumab and methotrexate achieved a 1.1 improvement from baseline in HAQ score at the end of 1 year, as compared with a 0.8 improvement in patients treated with methotrexate alone. With adalimumab alone, the improvement was 0.9.[21] In the light of these findings, it is not a surprise, but nonetheless very welcome, to see emerging data indicating that in early disease, treatment with infliximab and methotrexate gives a higher probability of maintaining employment than treatment with methotrexate alone.[31] These data would predict a lowering of the indirect costs associated with rheumatoid arthritis, such as disability benefits, as well as reduced direct costs of patient care over time, such as those associated with joint arthroplasty; but, as yet, there are few long-term data that can reliably offset the expense of anti-TNF therapies themselves against the anticipated long-term savings.

Safety of biological TNF inhibitors

In rheumatoid arthritis and many other chronic inflammatory diseases, many cellular and molecular processes contribute towards an immunological disequilibrium, in which normal homeostatic processes are unable to restore a healthy state and prevent the perpetuation of inflammatory processes. The success of TNF-α blockade in therapy suggests that this molecule occupies such a critical position in the pathogenic process. However, blockade of TNF or any other key physiological molecules may have the downside of negating their beneficial role in generating protective immune responses. For TNF-α antagonists, the key safety considerations include the following:

- infection, both common and opportunistic
- cytopenias
- demyelinating disease
- lupus-like syndromes

- congestive heart failure
- malignancies, particularly lymphomas.

There is now a considerable body of safety data for TNF inhibitors, and this has been obtained from various sources. They include information from placebo-controlled randomised clinical trials, post-drug approval databases, and long-term registries such as those established in the US, Sweden, Germany, and the UK. Despite the wealth of information available, there are a number of issues to consider when interpreting data about adverse events occurring during or after a period of anti-TNF treatment. For example, the patients recruited into clinical trials have to meet certain strict inclusion and exclusion criteria and, therefore, do not necessarily reflect the average patient attending a rheumatology department. Clinical trial populations may have a lower instance of co-morbidities, restricted usage of concomitant medication and, in some cases, a short exposure to the test drug during the period of the study. In the case of adverse-events data collected in the period following approval of the new agent, there is likely to be substantial under-reporting and the data are often incomplete and difficult to verify. It is often the case that serious adverse events are more likely to be reported than less serious events. A meaningful interpretation of post-approval events data ideally requires a comparator group of patients who are not treated with the new agent in order to determine to what extent the adverse event is likely to be attributable to the agent rather than to the disease itself or to concomitant therapies. In the case of some adverse events, in particular certain infectious complications, the data need to be interpreted in the light of the background rate of infection in the particular study population from which the data are captured.

Infectious complications

One of the most important and common safety concerns for the use of TNF inhibitors is the occurrence of infectious complications. In clinical trials, the rate of upper respiratory tract infections occurring in patients receiving TNF inhibitors, usually with concomitant methotrexate, is higher than that in patients receiving placebo injections or infusions together with methotrexate. However, the rate of serious infections has been consistently comparable between the groups receiving placebo and TNF inhibitor. Nonetheless, one of the most frequently occurring serious infections in the early days of anti-TNF treatment was mycobacterial tuberculosis, with extrapulmonary disease in about a third of cases. The incidence of complicating tuberculosis early in the history of infliximab therapy was about 1 in 1000 cases. However, the rate has substantially fallen since the introduction of screening programmes. Tuberculosis has been reported as a complication of all biological anti-TNF agents but with a varying prevalence, depending on the country in which the drug was used. Occurrence of complicating tuberculosis is strongly influenced by age, low socio-economic status, and geography. The background rate in the population is important, as the majority of cases of tuberculosis occurring following exposure to anti-TNF agents are thought to represent re-activation of latent tuberculosis. This may be because TNF blockade is a particularly effective way of breaking down granuloma walls. Where tuberculosis has been reported, the median time of onset in patients receiving etanercept is approximately 11 months, whereas 97% of patients reported as having tuberculosis following infliximab treatment developed the complication within 7 months.[32] Screening for and treating latent tuberculosis infection will prevent re-activation in most patients. Latent tuberculous infection screening should include a careful history including history of BCG vaccination, tuberculin skin test, and a chest radiograph. Skin testing is problematic, however, because of the occurrence of anergy in rheumatoid arthritis and high rate of false negative tuberculin skin tests as a consequence. Furthermore, for those inexperienced in skin testing, it is common to place injections or read the results inappropriately; therefore, training is required.

Because of the difficulties in interpreting tuberculin skin testing, there is now much interest in a newer generation of ELISPOT tests that are more sensitive, more specific, and more convenient than tuberculin skin tests. This test requires a single blood sample for the detection of IFN-γ- secreting T cells, with reactivity to peptides highly specific for latent mycobacterial tuberculosis infection.[33] However, the ELISPOT test is not yet widely available because it is costly and requires isolation of mononuclear cells, a procedure that is not performed in routine clinical laboratories.

Where latent tuberculosis is diagnosed or strongly suspected, prophylactic treatment should be offered in accordance with local guidelines and advice; for example, isoniazid for 9 months.[34] Although screening has greatly reduced the occurrence of mycobacterial tuberculosis with TNF antagonists, it has not been completely eliminated and there must always be a high degree of awareness for this and other granulomatous diseases.

A number of opportunistic infections have been reported with TNF inhibitors, both in the context of clinical trials and in adverse events reporting after drug approval. Although such infections are relatively rare, the most frequently occurring include histoplasmosis, *Pneumocystis carinii*, listeriosis and aspergillosis. The occurrence of these infections varies according to geographical location.

Because of the potential for infectious complications with TNF inhibitors, this class of drug is relatively contra-indicated in patients with chronic infectious states such as bronchiectasis or chronic sinusitis.

Congestive cardiac failure

Anti-TNF inhibitors must be used with great caution or avoided altogether in patients with a history of congestive cardiac failure. Although there have been theoretical arguments to support the potential benefits of TNF inhibition in this condition, clinical studies with both etanercept and infliximab failed to demonstrate

any benefit. Furthermore, in two clinical trials of etanercept in 2000 patients with moderate-to-severe cardiac failure (New York heart classification functional class 2–4), the findings suggested the possibility of increased mortality in patients receiving etanercept, in particular at a dose regimen of 3-times weekly. Infliximab has also been studied in a small group of patients with New York heart classification functional class 3 and 4 over a period of 1 year. In this study, there was an increased rate of hospitalisation and mortality in patients receiving infliximab at a dose of 10 mg/kg at baseline, week 2, and week 6.[35]

In a post-drug approval surveillance study, 47 patients treated with either etanercept or infliximab were identified as having congestive cardiac failure. Of these, 38 had new-onset disease and nine had exacerbations of prior disease.[36] There were no identifiable risk factors in half the patients with new onset heart failure, 29 of whom were treated with etanercept and 18 treated with infliximab. The onset of congestive cardiac failure ranged from 2 hours after treatment administration to 2 years, with a median time of 3.5 months. Ten patients under the age of 50 years developed new-onset congestive cardiac failure and three of these had pre-existing risk factors. The condition improved or resolved in nine of these ten patients after discontinuation of the TNF inhibitor and institution of therapy for congestive cardiac failure.

Solid tumours and lymphoma

Just as any powerful immunosuppressive agent raises concerns regarding infectious complications, similarly there are concerns that it may diminish immunosurveillance of abnormal cells and thus raise the risk of malignancy. However, the available data for all anti-TNF agents are re-assuring and suggest that the observed occurrence of non-haematological solid tumours in patients that have been exposed to TNF inhibitors is no different to that expected on the basis of frequencies in age-, sex-, and race-matched subjects from the surveillance, epidemiology, and end results (SEER database of the US National Cancer Institute).

Lymphomas of both Hodgkin's and non-Hodgkin's type have been reported as occurring in patients after exposure to all of the available TNF inhibitors, but it is difficult to ascribe an unequivocal causal link to the therapy. This is because rheumatoid arthritis itself is a risk factor for lymphoma, with a risk that correlates with the activity and severity of disease.[37] In one study, the odds ratio for development of lymphoma was 25.8 for rheumatoid patients with high inflammatory activity, compared with low inflammatory activity. The standardised incidence rates observed for lymphomas occurring with the use of TNF inhibitors in the context of clinical trials are within the range expected based on other publications for standardised incidence rates in rheumatoid arthritis itself. The contributions of other anti-rheumatic drugs to this risk, including azathioprine and methotrexate, are not clear. The majority of lymphomas observed with the use of TNF inhibitors are of non-Hodgkin's type, with a mean time to onset of 10–21 months.

In conclusion, there is a higher rate of lymphoma occurrence in rheumatoid patients than there is in healthy age- and sex-matched controls. Lymphomas have been reported in patients treated with anti-TNF therapies, but it remains unclear whether the medication is a contributory factor or causal or simply indicative of a patient population that is likely to have had more severe inflammatory disease activity prior to exposure to an anti-TNF drug.[35]

Other toxicity issues

New cases of central nervous system demyelination and exacerbations of pre-existing disease have been reported in patients with rheumatoid arthritis following exposure to TNF inhibitors. However, as in the case of lymphoma, any causal relationship remains controversial and unproven. In fact, TNF-α has been implicated in the pathogenesis of multiple sclerosis; because of this, there have been

studies of TNF inhibitors in this disease. In a Phase I open-label study, two patients with rapidly progressing multiple sclerosis refractory to high-dose intravenous corticosteroids were treated with intravenous infliximab. Both patients were found to have an increase in the number of gadalinium-enhancing lesions on MRI, together with increases in CSF leukocyte counts after each infusion. However, these changes were not accompanied by neurological deterioration.[38] In a Phase II multicentre study, 168 patients with relapsing–remitting and secondary progressive multiple sclerosis received monthly infusions of lenercept (a recombinant soluble TNF p55 receptor fusion protein) at 3 dose levels or placebo for up to 48 weeks. Although this treatment was not associated with an increase in the number of new lesions, on MRI scanning it was sufficiently associated with increased demyelination attack frequency but not duration or severity.[39] Neurological events associated with demyelinating lesions on MRI have been reported in patients treated with anti-TNF agents.[40] However, the rate of new cases of multiple sclerosis reported in post-marketing surveillance for infliximab, etanercept, and adalimumab is at, or below, the number of expected cases based on the background rate for society as a whole, which is approximately 6 new cases per 100,000 per year.[41] Although there is no proven relationship between TNF inhibition and onset of a demyelinating episode, it is wisest to avoid TNF inhibitors in patients with a history of optic neuritis, transverse myelitis, or other form of CNS demyelination.

In clinical trial data, induction of anti-nuclear antibodies and antibodies to double-stranded DNA have been reported with higher frequency in patients receiving TNF inhibitors than in comparator groups not receiving these drugs. Although induction of antibodies to double-stranded DNA is relatively common, in the order of 10–15% of patients, the occurrence of clinical features of SLE is much less common. Sulphasalazine, widely used in the treatment of rheumatoid arthritis, is also associated with a similar pattern of autoantibody induction. In reported cases of clinical lupus following exposure to TNF inhibitors, the onset of symptoms occurs 1.5–18 months after introduction of the anti-TNF agent, with a mean time of 4.4 months, and women are predominantly affected. The syndrome abates on cessation of the TNF inhibitor and introduction of corticosteroid therapy as appropriate.[42]

Injection site reactions or infusion-related reactions

Safety issues involving the anti-TNF agents as a class include the risk of injection site reactions or infusion-related reactions. These are usually mild, however, and most often easily managed. For example, in the case of the self-administered subcutaneous delivery of etanercept, injection site reactions were reported in 37% of etanercept-treated patients versus 10% of controls in placebo-controlled trials. These reactions are generally mild-to-moderate, occur sporadically in a minority of injections over time, and do not necessitate the discontinuation of the agent. Similarly, in the case of adalimumab, which is also given by self-administered subcutaneous injection, injection site reactions are the most commonly reported adverse event, occurring in 19.5% of treated patients versus 11.6% of controls. Reactions may take the form of erythema, itching, haemorrhage, pain, or swelling at the injection site, although such events very rarely merit the discontinuation of the therapy. In the case of infliximab, infusion-related reactions may occur within one to two hours of the infusion itself. In clinical trial data, 22% of infliximab-treated patients experienced an infusion reaction compared with 9% of controls. However, it is also the case from clinical trial data that less than 5% of infliximab infusions are associated with infusion reactions, compared with 2% of placebo infusions. Fewer than 1% of infliximab-treated patients develop serious infusion reactions and it is rarely necessary to discontinue therapy. Most infusion-related

reactions are mild and non-specific and may simply require slowing of the infusion rate and administration of paracetamol and/or an antihistamine. Similarly, symptomatic injection site reactions with etanercept or adalimumab can be managed with local warm compresses and oral antihistamines if required.

Mechanism of action of TNF blockade

> **Learning point**
>
> Putative mechanisms of action of TNF inhibitors
>
> - de-activation of the pro-inflammatory cytokine cascade at the site of inflammation
> - reduction in mediators of joint destruction
> - diminished recruitment of inflammatory cells from the blood to the rheumatoid joint
> - diminished synovial vascularity
> - a role in modulation of apoptosis remains controversial

A number of mechanisms of action of TNF inhibitors have been identified to date. These include: de-activation of the pro-inflammatory cytokine cascade at the site of inflammation; reduction in mediators of joint destruction; diminished recruitment of inflammatory cells from the blood to the rheumatoid joint and diminished synovial vascularity (Fig. 7.2). A role in modulation of apoptosis remains controversial.

The first formal proof that TNF-α regulates other pro-inflammatory cytokines *in vivo* was the observation that there is a rapid reduction in serum IL-6 concentrations, closely followed by falling serum CRP, following administration of infliximab.[43,44] Although IL-1 concentrations are often below the limit of detection in the peripheral blood of rheumatoid arthritis patients, where it is detectable, down-regulation has been reported in a proportion of patients.[45] Similarly, in a small study of repeat synovial biopsies obtained before and 2 weeks after a single infusion of 10 mg/kg of infliximab, computerised image analysis of

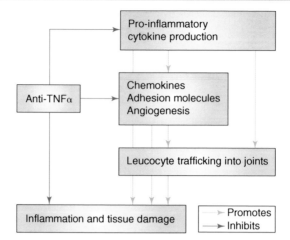

Figure 7.2
Mechanisms of action of biological TNF-α inhibitors

sections stained for cytokine-producing cells demonstrated a reduction in synovial IL-1α and IL-1β in a subgroup.[46] It is clear that the benefits of anti-TNF therapy are not mediated by up-regulation of endogenous pro-inflammatory cytokine inhibitors, since circulating IL-1ra and soluble TNF receptor levels fall after infliximab infusion.[44]

It is thought that a major mechanism of action of TNF inhibitors is likely to be mediated by modulation of inflammatory cell traffic. A dose-dependent rise in peripheral blood lymphocyte counts is observed following infliximab infusion, with a maximum rise within 24 hours of treatment.[47] This is mediated by modulation of both arms of the inflammatory cell recruitment cascade. Thus, there is reduced histological expression of synovial cytokine-induced vascular adhesion molecules, such as E-selectin and VCAM-1, following anti-TNF treatment[48] and a significant dose-dependent reduction in soluble serum E-selectin and ICAM-1 concentrations,[47] as well as significantly diminished immunohistological expression of the chemokines IL-8 and MCP-1, with a trend to reduction in a number of other chemokines.[49]

Further indirect evidence to suggest TNF blockade reduces inflammatory cell recruitment

to the joint is based on the observation that infliximab therapy is associated with a reduction in numbers of synovial tissue macrophages and lymphocytes.[48,49] However, the definitive confirmation that TNF-α blockade reduces leukocyte traffic to inflamed joints was obtained in an open-label clinical trial demonstrating a 40–50% decrease in retention of autologous indium-111 labelled granulocytes in the hands, wrists, and knees 2 weeks after infliximab treatment.[49] There is a reduction in the marginating granulocyte pool after infliximab treatment, an observation that would normally be associated with a rise in peripheral blood granulocyte counts.[50] However, in contrast to peripheral blood lymphocyte counts, numbers of peripheral blood granulocytes decrease after infliximab with maximal changes within 24 hours. The reason for this is that myeloid cell production is reduced secondary to down-regulation of GM-CSF as a consequence of TNF blockade. Because of the short circulating half-life of the granulocyte, of approximately 8 hours, a diminished rate of cell production dominates the peripheral blood picture.

One factor contributing to the very rapid reduction in joint swelling observed by both patients and physicians after anti-TNF therapy is likely to be a reduction in tissue oedema and capillary leak, mediated by vascular endothelial growth factor (VEGF), a cytokine implicated in new blood vessel formation and found to be elevated in the serum of rheumatoid arthritis patients.[51] Serum concentrations of VEGF show a dose-dependent reduction following infliximab infusions, but without normalisation. There is also reduction in synovial vascular density and, in particular, a reduction in angiogenesis, as assessed by diminished expression of vessels expressed the $\alpha_V\beta_3$ integrin.[52] Further evidence for a reduction in synovial vascularity following TNF blockade is the observation that the vascular signal on quantitative power Doppler imaging is significantly reduced following infliximab therapy.[53,54]

Relatively early in the history of clinical trials of TNF blockade, marked reduction in circulating concentrations of the precursors of the matrix metalloproteinase enzymes MMP-1 and MMP-3 were reported[55] as well as a significant reduction in synovial tissue expression of matrix metalloproteinases.[56] Similarly, serum levels of osteoprotegerin (OPG) and soluble receptor activator of nuclear factor κB ligands (sRANKL), both of which are elevated in rheumatoid compared to normal sera, are normalised following infliximab therapy without influencing the OPG:sRankL ratio.[57] These observations predicted the disease-modifying capability of anti-TNF inhibitors, which is now established.

One hypothesis for the failure of the p75 TNF receptor fusion protein etanercept to give clinical benefits in trials of Crohn's disease, in contrast to the marked benefits demonstrated with monoclonal antibodies to TNF-α, is that the antibodies may cause an increase in apoptosis of lamina propria and peripheral T cells through caspase-dependent mechanisms.[58] However, this topic remains controversial and the relevance of modulation of apoptosis as the mechanism of action of TNF inhibitors in rheumatoid arthritis is unclear. In one study, decreased synovial cellularity was reported as early as 48 hours after infliximab administration, but with no corresponding

evidence of apoptosis.[59] In another study, however, apoptosis in synovial macrophages has been reported to be induced by both etanercept and infliximab, with a corresponding increase in active caspase-3 expression. No increase in lymphocyte apoptosis was observed, however.[60] The relevance of these interesting observations to the mode of action of TNF inhibitors in rheumatoid arthritis is not clear.

Biological therapies targeting IL-1

Studies in animal models of arthritis have demonstrated the therapeutic potential of IL-1 blockade.[61] The dominance of IL-1β over IL-1α in the pathogenesis of collagen-induced arthritis has been demonstrated in studies of cytokine blockade[62,63] and confirmed by the finding that IL-1β gene knock-out mice show markedly reduced levels of inflammation following immunisation with type II collagen. The use of genetically modified mice has also helped to confirm the physiological significance of IL-1ra as deletion of this gene in BALB/c mice results in the spontaneous development of arthritis.[64]

Proof of principle for IL-1 blockade in rheumatoid arthritis has been established using once-daily, subcutaneously-administered IL-1 receptor antagonist (IL-1ra: anakinra), a naturally occurring inhibitor of IL-1 (Fig. 7.3).[65] In a phase II placebo-controlled study, 472 patients received daily subcutaneous injections of placebo or one of three different doses of human IL-1ra – 30 mg, 75 mg, or 150 mg. Improvements were observed in all individual clinical parameters, including swollen and tender joint counts, pain score, duration of early morning stiffness, patient assessment of disease activity, and investigator assessment of disease activity, although no clear dose–response relationship was observed. At the end of the study period, significantly more patients on the higher dosage schedule achieved improvement at the ACR 20% response level than placebo-treated patients. There were also significant reductions in ESR in all active treatment groups. However, the overall

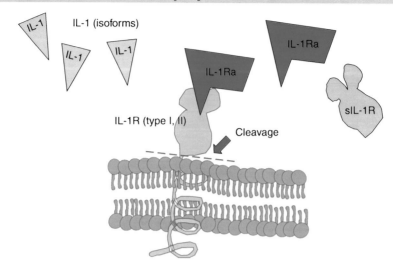

Figure 7.3
IL-1 receptor antagonist. Adapted from Moreland *et al.*[68] Reprinted with permission of Wiley–Liss, Inc., a subsidiary of John Wiley & Sons, Inc. © 1997, John Wiley & Sons, Inc.

magnitude of clinical responses and changes in acute phase reactants were relatively modest, at 20–35% from baseline, as compared with those reported for TNF-α blockade. These observations do not necessarily imply that IL-1 is not a good target for therapy in rheumatoid arthritis, but may reflect pharmacokinetic challenges for IL-1ra as a means to achieve IL-1 blockade. For example, the kidneys excrete IL-1ra rapidly and therapeutic levels persist for a few hours only. Furthermore, IL-1 receptors are ubiquitously expressed and have a rapid turnover. Nonetheless, daily administration of human IL-1ra has been reported to have the benefit of disease modification, with a reduction in the rate of radiographic damage in patients receiving active drug as compared with those on placebo. However, the reduction only reached statistical significance in patients receiving the two lower doses.

The efficacy and safety of anakinra in combination with methotrexate has been tested in a multicentre, randomised, double-blind, placebo-controlled trial.[66] In this study, patients with moderate to severely active rheumatoid arthritis despite methotrexate therapy for 6 consecutive months, with stable

doses for more than 3 months, were randomised to receive either single daily placebo injections or one of five different doses of anakinra. At week 12, the ACR 20 responses in the five active treatment plus methotrexate groups demonstrated a statistically significant dose–response relationship over that in the placebo plus methotrexate group, and these responses endured through 24 weeks. The combination of anakinra and methotrexate was safe and well tolerated.

Although IL-1 blockade using anakinra in combination with methotrexate has been shown to be clinically superior to methotrexate therapy alone, the disappointing magnitude of clinical efficacy as compared with that seen with TNF inhibitors has prompted the exploration of alternative strategies for exploring IL-1. These include the use of monoclonal antibodies with specificity for IL-1β, and the IL-1 trap, an engineered protein comprising the two high-affinity signalling chains of the cell surface IL-1 receptor, linked by the Fc portion of IgG$_1$. Preliminary results presented at meetings demonstrate efficacy for the IL-1 trap at the higher dose tested.

Combination anti-cytokine therapies

The wide-spread use of conventional DMARDs in combination with an apparent increase in efficacy without raising significant regards concerning toxicity or tolerability has prompted the investigation of combination anti-cytokine therapy.[67] The potential attractions of this approach include superior immunomodulation and hence enhanced efficacy. However, in a 24-week randomised controlled trial conducted in 242 patients with rheumatoid arthritis who had not previously been treated with biological agents and were taking background methotrexate, the combination of etanercept 25 mg twice weekly together with anakinra 100 mg once daily resulted in an incidence of serious infection of 7% and the occurrence of neutropenia in the combination group. The incidence of both infection and neutropenia was higher in the combination group than in the Enbrel alone group and higher than the rate observed in studies using anakinra alone. Furthermore, there was no therapeutic benefit of the combination treatment over etanercept alone. For this reason, the concomitant use of IL-1 blockade and TNF inhibitors is not recommended.[67]

Conclusions

The anti-TNF agents have been demonstrated to provide a marked improvement in outcomes in a proportion of patients with rheumatoid arthritis. Furthermore, they are well tolerated. Injection site reactions or infusion-related reactions are relatively common but easily managed and rarely lead to discontinuation of therapy. These drugs do lead to an increased incidence of upper respiratory tract infections and more rarely to serious opportunistic or tuberculous infections. With appropriate screening, some infections can be prevented and those that do occur generally respond to appropriate medical treatment. However, it is important to emphasise the value of screening, education, and monitoring of patients. There is no established causal relationship between exposure to anti-TNF agents and the occurrence of demyelinating disorders or malignancies; nonetheless, cases have been reported and, therefore, vigilance is necessary. Overall, the anti-TNF biologicals have demonstrated a risk–benefit profile that markedly favours an overall benefit.

References

1. Scallon B, Cai A, Solowski N et al. Binding and functional comparisons of two types of tumor necrosis factor antagonists. J Pharmacol Exp Ther 2002; **301**: 418–26.

2. Hazleman B, Smith M, Moss K et al. Efficacy of a novel pegylated humanised anti-TNF fragment (CDP870) in patients with rheumatoid arthritis. Rheumatology 2000; **39 (Suppl 1)**: 87.

3. Maini RN, Taylor PC. Anti-cytokine therapy in rheumatoid arthritis. Annu Rev Med 2000; **51**: 207–29.

4. Brennan FM, Chantry D, Jackson A, Maini R, Feldmann M. Inhibitory effect of TNF alpha antibodies on synovial cell interleukin-1 production in rheumatoid arthritis. Lancet 1989; **2**: 244–7.

5. Butler DM, Maini RN, Feldmann M, Brennan FM. Modulation of pro-inflammatory cytokine release in rheumatoid synovial membrane cell cultures. Comparison of monoclonal anti TNF-alpha antibody with the interleukin-1 receptor antagonist. Eur Cytokine Netw 1995; **6**: 225–30.

6. Haworth C, Brennan FM, Chantry D, Turner M, Maini RN, Feldmann M. Expression of granulocyte-macrophage colony-stimulating factor in rheumatoid arthritis: regulation by tumor necrosis factor-alpha. Eur J Immunol 1991; **21**: 2575–9.

7. Williams RO, Feldmann M, Maini RN. Cartilage destruction and bone erosion in arthritis: the role of tumour necrosis factor alpha. Ann Rheum Dis 2000; **59 (Suppl 1)**:i75–80.

8. Keffer J, Probert L, Cazlaris H et al. Transgenic mice expressing human tumour necrosis factor: a predictive genetic model of arthritis. EMBO J 1991; **10**: 4025–31.

9. Buchan G, Barrett K, Turner M, Chantry D, Maini RN, Feldmann M. Interleukin-1 and tumour necrosis factor mRNA expression in rheumatoid arthritis: prolonged production of IL-1 alpha. Clin Exp Immunol 1988; **73**: 449–55.

10. Dayer JM, Beutler B, Cerami A. Cachectin/tumor necrosis factor stimulates collagenase and prostaglandin E_2 production by human synovial cells and dermal fibroblasts. J Exp Med 1985; **162**: 2163–8.

11. Williams RO, Feldmann M, Maini RN. Anti-tumor necrosis factor ameliorates joint disease in murine collagen-induced arthritis. Proc Natl Acad Sci USA 1992; **89**: 9784–8.

12. Piguet PF, Grau GE, Vesin C, Loetscher H, Gentz R, Lesslauer W. Evolution of collagen arthritis in mice is arrested by treatment with anti-tumour necrosis factor (TNF) antibody or a recombinant soluble TNF receptor. *Immunology* 1992; **77**: 510–4.

13. Elliott MJ, Maini RN, Feldmann M *et al.* Treatment of rheumatoid arthritis with chimeric monoclonal antibodies to tumor necrosis factor alpha. *Arthritis Rheum* 1993; **36**: 1681–90.

14. Kremer JM, Weinblatt ME, Bankhurst AD *et al.* Etanercept added to background methotrexate therapy in patients with rheumatoid arthritis: continued observations. *Arthritis Rheum* 2003; **48**: 1493–9.

15. Maini RN, Breedveld FC, Kalden JR *et al.* and Anti-Tumor Necrosis Factor Trial in Rheumatoid Arthritis with Concomitant Therapy Study Group. Sustained improvement over two years in physical function, structural damage, and signs and symptoms among patients with rheumatoid arthritis treated with infliximab and methotrexate. *Arthritis Rheum.* 2004; **50**: 1051–65.

16. Lipsky PE, van der Heijde DM, St Clair EW *et al.* and Anti-Tumor Necrosis Factor Trial in Rheumatoid Arthritis with Concomitant Therapy Study Group. Infliximab and methotrexate in the treatment of rheumatoid arthritis. Anti-Tumor Necrosis Factor Trial in Rheumatoid Arthritis with Concomitant Therapy Study Group. *N Engl J Med* 2000; **343**: 1594–602.

17. Klareskog L, van der Heijde D, de Jager JP *et al.* and TEMPO (Trial of Etanercept and Methotrexate with Radiographic Patient Outcomes) study investigators. Therapeutic effect of the combination of etanercept and methotrexate compared with each treatment alone in patients with rheumatoid arthritis: double-blind randomised controlled trial. *Lancet* 2004; **363**: 675–81.

18. St Clair EW, van der Heijde DM, Smolen JS *et al.* and Active-Controlled Study of Patients Receiving Infliximab for the Treatment of Rheumatoid Arthritis of Early Onset Study Group. Combination of infliximab and methotrexate therapy for early rheumatoid arthritis: a randomized, controlled trial. *Arthritis Rheum* 2004; **50**: 3432–43.

19. Breedveld FC, Emery P, Keystone E *et al.* Infliximab in active early rheumatoid arthritis. *Ann Rheum Dis* 2004; **63**: 149–55.

20. Emery P. Adalimumab therapy: clinical findings and implications for integration into clinical guidelines for rheumatoid arthritis. *Drugs Today (Barc)* 2005; **41**: 155–63.

21. Breedveld FC, Weisman MH, Kavanaugh AF *et al.* The PREMIER study: a multicenter, randomized, double-blind clinical trial of combination therapy with adalimumab plus methotrexate versus methotrexate alone or adalimumab alone in patients with early, aggressive rheumatoid arthritis who had not had previous methotrexate treatment. *Arthritis Rheum* 2006; **54**: 26–37.

22. Bathon JM, Martin RW, Fleischmann RM *et al.* A comparison of etanercept and methotrexate in patients with early rheumatoid arthritis. *N Engl J Med* 2000; **343**: 1586–93. Erratum in: *N Engl J Med* 2001; **344**: 240 and *N Engl J Med* 2001; **344**: 76.

23. Genovese MC, Bathon JM, Martin RW *et al.* Etanercept versus methotrexate in patients with early rheumatoid arthritis: two-year radiographic and clinical outcomes. *Arthritis Rheum* 2002; **46**: 1443–50.

24. Weinblatt ME, Kremer JM, Bankhurst AD *et al.* A trial of etanercept, a recombinant tumor necrosis factor receptor:Fc fusion protein, in patients with rheumatoid arthritis receiving methotrexate. *N Engl J Med* 1999; **340**: 253–9.

25. Maini R, St Clair EW, Breedveld F *et al.* Infliximab (chimeric anti-tumour necrosis factor alpha monoclonal antibody) versus placebo in rheumatoid arthritis patients receiving concomitant methotrexate: a randomised phase III trial. ATTRACT Study Group. *Lancet* 1999; **354**: 1932–9.

26. Keystone EC, Kavanaugh AF, Sharp JT *et al.* Radiographic, clinical, and functional outcomes of treatment with adalimumab (a human anti-tumor necrosis factor monoclonal antibody) in patients with active rheumatoid arthritis receiving concomitant methotrexate therapy: a randomized, placebo-controlled, 52-week trial. *Arthritis Rheum* 2004; **50**: 1400–11.

27. Maini RN, Breedveld FC, Kalden JR *et al.* Therapeutic efficacy of multiple intravenous infusions of anti-tumor necrosis factor alpha monoclonal antibody combined with low-dose weekly methotrexate in rheumatoid arthritis. *Arthritis Rheum* 1998; **41**: 1552–63.

28. Brennan FM, Browne KA, Green PA, Jaspar JM, Maini RN, Feldmann M. Reduction of serum matrix metalloproteinase 1 and matrix metalloproteinase 3 in rheumatoid arthritis patients following anti-tumour necrosis factor-alpha (cA2) therapy. *Br J Rheumatol* 1997; **36**: 643–50.

29. Smolen JS, Han C, Bala M *et al.* and ATTRACT Study Group. Evidence of radiographic benefit of treatment with infliximab plus methotrexate in rheumatoid arthritis patients who had no clinical improvement: a detailed subanalysis of data from the anti-tumor necrosis factor trial in rheumatoid arthritis with concomitant therapy study. *Arthritis Rheum* 2005; **52**: 1020–30.

30. Maini RN, Breedveld FC, Kalden JR *et al.* and Anti-Tumor Necrosis Factor Trial in Rheumatoid Arthritis with Concomitant Therapy Study Group. Sustained improvement over two years in physical function, structural damage, and signs and symptoms among patients with rheumatoid arthritis treated with infliximab and methotrexate. *Arthritis Rheum* 2004; **50**: 1051–65.

31. Smolen JS, Han C, van der Heijde D *et al.* Infliximab treatment maintains employability in patients with early rheumatoid arthritis. *Arthritis Rheum* 2006; **54**: 716–22.

32. Keane J, Gershon S, Wise RP et al. Tuberculosis associated with infliximab, a tumor necrosis factor alpha-neutralizing agent. *N Engl J Med* 2001; **345**: 1098–104.

33. Lalvani A, Nagvenkar P, Udwadia Z et al. Enumeration of T cells specific for RD1-encoded antigens suggests a high prevalence of latent *Mycobacterium tuberculosis* infection in healthy urban Indians. *J Infect Dis* 2001; **183**: 469–77.

34. Keane J. TNF-blocking agents and tuberculosis: new drugs illuminate an old topic. *Rheumatology (Oxford)* 2005; **44**: 714–20.

35. Keystone EC. Advances in targeted therapy: safety of biological agents. *Ann Rheum Dis* 2003; **62 (Suppl 2)**: ii34–6.

36. Kwon HJ, Cote TR, Cuffe MS, Kramer JM, Braun MM. Case reports of heart failure after therapy with a tumor necrosis factor antagonist. *Ann Intern Med* 2003; **138**: 807–11.

37. Baecklund E, Ekbom A, Sparen P, Feltelius N, Klareskog L. Disease activity and risk of lymphoma in patients with rheumatoid arthritis: nested case-control study. *BMJ* 1998; **317**: 180–1.

38. van Oosten BW, Barkhof F, Truyen L et al. Increased MRI activity and immune activation in two multiple sclerosis patients treated with the monoclonal anti-tumor necrosis factor antibody cA2. *Neurology* 1996; **47**: 1531–4.

39. Klinkert WE, Kojima K, Lesslauer W, Rinner W, Lassmann H, Wekerle H. TNF-alpha receptor fusion protein prevents experimental auto-immune encephalomyelitis and demyelination in Lewis rats: an overview. *J Neuroimmunol* 1997; **72**: 163–8.

40. Mohan N, Edwards ET, Cupps TR et al. Demyelination occurring during anti-tumor necrosis factor alpha therapy for inflammatory arthritides. *Arthritis Rheum* 2001; **44**: 2862–9.

41. Noseworthy JH, Lucchinetti C, Rodriguez M, Weinshenker BG. Multiple sclerosis. *N Engl J Med* 2000; **343**: 938–52.

42. Mohan AK, Edwards ET, Cote TR, Siegel JN, Braun MM. Drug-induced systemic lupus erythematosus and TNF-alpha blockers. *Lancet* 2002; **360**: 646.

43. Elliott MJ, Maini RN, Feldmann M et al. Repeated therapy with monoclonal antibody to tumour necrosis factor alpha (cA2) in patients with rheumatoid arthritis. *Lancet* 1994; **344**: 1125–7.

44. Charles P, Elliott MJ, Davis D et al. Regulation of cytokines, cytokine inhibitors, and acute-phase proteins following anti-TNF-alpha therapy in rheumatoid arthritis. *J Immunol* 1999; **163**: 1521–8.

45. Lorenz HM, Antoni C, Valerius T et al. *In vivo* blockade of TNF-alpha by intravenous infusion of a chimeric monoclonal TNF-alpha antibody in patients with rheumatoid arthritis. Short term cellular and molecular effects. *J Immunol* 1996; **156**: 1646–53.

46. Ulfgren AK, Andersson U, Engstrom M, Klareskog L, Maini RN, Taylor PC. Systemic anti-tumor necrosis factor alpha therapy in rheumatoid arthritis down-regulates synovial tumor necrosis factor alpha synthesis. *Arthritis Rheum* 2000; **43**: 2391–6.

47. Paleolog EM, Hunt M, Elliott MJ, Feldmann M, Maini RN, Woody JN. Deactivation of vascular endothelium by monoclonal anti-tumor necrosis factor alpha antibody in rheumatoid arthritis. *Arthritis Rheum* 1996; **39**: 1082–91.

48. Tak PP, Taylor PC, Breedveld FC et al. Decrease in cellularity and expression of adhesion molecules by anti-tumor necrosis factor alpha monoclonal antibody treatment in patients with rheumatoid arthritis. *Arthritis Rheum* 1996; **39**: 1077–81.

49. Taylor PC, Peters AM, Paleolog E et al. Reduction of chemokine levels and leukocyte traffic to joints by tumor necrosis factor alpha blockade in patients with rheumatoid arthritis. *Arthritis Rheum* 2000; **43**: 38–47.

50. Taylor PC, Peters AM, Glass DM, Maini RN. Effects of treatment of rheumatoid arthritis patients with an antibody against tumour necrosis factor alpha on reticuloendothelial and intrapulmonary granulocyte traffic. *Clin Sci (Lond)* 1999; **97**: 85–9.

51. Paleolog EM, Young S, Stark AC, McCloskey RV, Feldmann M, Maini RN. Modulation of angiogenic vascular endothelial growth factor by tumor necrosis factor alpha and interleukin-1 in rheumatoid arthritis. *Arthritis Rheum* 1998; **41**: 1258–65.

52. Taylor PC. Serum vascular markers and vascular imaging in assessment of rheumatoid arthritis disease activity and response to therapy. *Rheumatology (Oxford)* 2005; **44**: 721–8.

53. Taylor PC, Steuer A, Gruber J et al. Comparison of ultrasonographic assessment of synovitis and joint vascularity with radiographic evaluation in a randomized, placebo-controlled study of infliximab therapy in early rheumatoid arthritis. *Arthritis Rheum* 2004; **50**: 1107–16.

54. Taylor PC, Steuer A, Gruber J et al. Ultrasonographic and radiographic results from a two-year controlled trial of immediate or one-year-delayed addition of infliximab to ongoing methotrexate therapy in patients with erosive early rheumatoid arthritis. *Arthritis Rheum* 2006; **54**: 47–53.

55. Brennan FM, Browne KA, Green PA, Jaspar JM, Maini RN, Feldmann M. Reduction of serum matrix metalloproteinase 1 and matrix metallo-proteinase 3 in rheumatoid arthritis patients following anti-tumour necrosis factor-alpha (cA2) therapy. *Br J Rheumatol* 1997; **36**: 643–50.

56. Catrina AI, Lampa J, Ernestam S et al. Anti-tumour necrosis factor (TNF)-alpha therapy (etanercept) down-regulates serum matrix metalloproteinase (MMP)-3 and MMP-1 in rheumatoid arthritis. *Rheumatology (Oxford)* 2002; **41**: 484–9.

57. Ziolkowska M, Kurowska M, Radzikowska A et al. High levels of osteoprotegerin and soluble receptor activator of nuclear factor kappa B ligand in serum of rheumatoid arthritis patients and their normalization after anti-tumor necrosis factor alpha treatment. *Arthritis Rheum* 2002; **46**: 1744–53.

58. Van den Brande JM, Braat H, van den Brink GR *et al.* Infliximab but not etanercept induces apoptosis in lamina propria T-lymphocytes from patients with Crohn's disease. *Gastroenterology* 2003; **124**: 1774–85.

59. Smeets TJ, Kraan MC, van Loon ME, Tak PP. Tumor necrosis factor alpha blockade reduces the synovial cell infiltrate early after initiation of treatment, but apparently not by induction of apoptosis in synovial tissue. *Arthritis Rheum* 2003; **48**: 2155–62.

60. Catrina AI, Trollmo C, af Klint E *et al.* Evidence that anti-tumor necrosis factor therapy with both etanercept and infliximab induces apoptosis in macrophages, but not lymphocytes, in rheumatoid arthritis joints: extended report. *Arthritis Rheum* 2005; **52**: 61–72.

61. van den Berg WB. Arguments for interleukin 1 as a target in chronic arthritis. *Ann Rheum Dis* 2000; **59 (Suppl 1)**: i81–4.

62. Joosten LA, Helsen MM, van de Loo FA, van den Berg WB. Anticytokine treatment of established type II collagen-induced arthritis in DBA/1 mice. A comparative study using anti-TNF alpha, anti-IL-1 alpha/beta, and IL-1Ra. *Arthritis Rheum* 1996; **39**: 797–809.

63. Williams RO, Marinova-Mutafchieva L, Feldmann M, Maini RN. Evaluation of TNF-alpha and IL-1 blockade in collagen-induced arthritis and comparison with combined anti-TNF-alpha/anti-CD4 therapy. *J Immunol* 2000; **165**: 7240–5.

64. Horai R, Saijo S, Tanioka H *et al.* Development of chronic inflammatory arthropathy resembling rheumatoid arthritis in interleukin 1 receptor antagonist-deficient mice. *J Exp Med* 2000; **191**: 313–20.

65. Bresnihan B, Alvaro-Gracia JM, Cobby M *et al.* Treatment of rheumatoid arthritis with recombinant human interleukin-1 receptor antagonist. *Arthritis Rheum.* 1998; **41**: 2196–204.

66. Cohen S, Hurd E, Cush J *et al.* Treatment of rheumatoid arthritis with anakinra, a recombinant human interleukin-1 receptor antagonist, in combination with methotrexate: results of a twenty-four-week, multicenter, randomized, double-blind, placebo-controlled trial. *Arthritis Rheum* 2002; **46**: 614–24.

67. Genovese MC, Cohen S, Moreland L *et al.* and 20000223 Study Group. Combination therapy with etanercept and anakinra in the treatment of patients with rheumatoid arthritis who have been treated unsuccessfully with methotrexate. *Arthritis Rheum* 2004; **50**: 1412–9.

68. Moreland LW, Heck LW Jr, Koopman WT. Biologic agents for treating rheumatoid arthritis. Concepts and progress. *Arthritis Rheum* 1997; **40**: 397–409.

8 Rationale for a new paradigm in pharmacotherapeutics for rheumatoid arthritis

Joint destruction occurs early in arthritis

A window of opportunity

Optimising suppression of synovitis in early rheumatoid arthritis

Conclusions

The majority of physicians who trained more than a decade ago would have been taught that non-steroidal anti-inflammatory drugs (NSAIDs) were the first-line treatment for rheumatoid arthritis, and that so-called disease-modifying anti-rheumatic drugs (DMARDs) available at the time, including gold, penicillamine, methotrexate, sulphasalazine, and hydroxychloroquine, were to be introduced later on in the established phase of disease once signs of joint deformity became evident. This teaching was based on the concept that NSAIDs have relatively little toxicity as compared with DMARDs and that the DMARDs had relatively little effect on joint destruction. However, this approach to the pharmacotherapeutics for rheumatoid arthritis has been entirely discredited for a number of reasons. First, it is not the case that NSAIDs are without toxicities, as discussed in detail in chapter 6. Second, in the last decade or so, it has clearly emerged that early and optimum suppression of synovitis with DMARDs leads to a much more favourable outcome in terms of inhibition of structural damage to joints and

overall well-being. Furthermore, with an appropriate drug monitoring programme, the toxicities associated with DMARDs can be greatly reduced.

> **Learning points**
>
> - The teaching that patients with rheumatoid arthritis should be treated with NSAIDs along at presentation, with late introduction of DMARDs, is now discredited.
>
> - If a patient presenting to a primary care practitioner with polyarthritis responds well to an NSAID, this is not a reason to delay referral and such patients often have an excellent outcome with early introduction of DMARDs.
>
> - The majority of patients presenting with rheumatoid arthritis will require treatment with NSAIDs for symptomatic benefit, in addition to DMARDs both for suppression of synovitis and inhibition of structural damage.
>
> - NSAIDs have two actions: they are analgesic and anti-inflammatory. However, they have no effect whatsoever on the destructive phase of disease responsible for progressive structural damage to joints.
>
> - If rheumatoid arthritis patients taking DMARDs still require high NSAID doses, it may indicate that better control of synovitis is required with a higher DMARD dose.

Joint destruction occurs early in arthritis

There is considerable evidence that radiographic damage, loss of function,[1] and loss of bone mineral density[2] occur very early in the disease process (Fig. 8.1). For example, it has been reported that in early rheumatoid arthritis of less than 6 months' symptom duration, up to 40% of patients have erosive disease at presentation:[3] similarly, by magnetic resonance imaging (MRI), bone marrow oedema can be detected within 4 weeks of symptom onset.[4] In another study of 42 patients with early phase rheumatoid arthritis, with symptom duration of only 4 months, MRI scans were evaluated using validated methods by two musculoskeletal

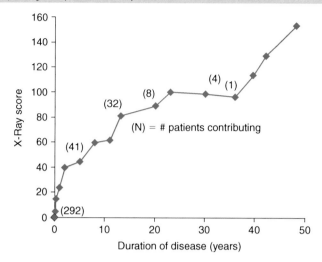

Figure 8.1
Erosions and cartilage destruction are nearly universal features in peripheral joints that have been chronically affected by rheumatoid arthritis. In this study, the investigators examined 292 patients. The average annual rate of progression of the total radiological score, which sums erosion and joint space abnormalities and has a maximum possible score of 314, was approximately 4 units per year over the first 25 years after onset. The progression of damage was more rapid in the early years and slightly slower in the later years. Adapted from Sharp *et al.*[23] with permission of Wiley–Liss, Inc., a subsidiary of John Wiley & Sons, Inc. © 1991 John Wiley & Sons.

radiologists, and were compared with plain radiographs. Erosions were detected in 45% of the MRI scans and 15% of the radiographs.[5] In this patient population, bone marrow oedema was detected in 64% of patients, synovitis in 93%, and tendonitis in 79%.

In a report summarising prospective studies using conventional radiography to assess progression of joint damage in early rheumatoid arthritis, it was concluded that about 75% of patients developed erosions within the first 2 years of symptom onset.[6] In a prospective study of 147 patients with early rheumatoid arthritis followed over 2 years, of which 90 patients were followed over 3 years, the rate of progression in the first year was found to be significantly higher than in the second and third years. Of the 90 patients followed for 3 years, 70% showed radiographic damage that could be identified one year after diagnosis. Overall, after 3 years, approximately 20% of the joints were affected.[6] These studies indicate that the rate of progression of structural

damage to joints is rapid in the early stages of rheumatoid disease, and emphasise the importance of initiating therapy with the potential to retard or stop this damage at the earliest time point. At the present time, once established, bone destruction cannot be reversed.

A window of opportunity: evidence to support improved radiographic outcomes with optimal suppression of synovitis in the earliest stages of disease

Comparing the timing of treatment initiation and its impact on disease progression

In 1995, Egsmose *et al.*[7] published the results of a 5-year follow-up study in which early treatment with intramuscular gold was compared with a delayed treatment strategy. The early treatment group showed superior improvement with respect to symptoms and signs, physical function, and joint damage, supporting the hypothesis that there is a therapeutic window of opportunity early in the disease course. In 1996, the results of a randomised controlled trial comparing immediate and delayed introduction of DMARD therapy in patients with recently diagnosed rheumatoid arthritis were published. Similarly, outcomes including inhibition of joint damage were improved in those patients treated with early DMARD introduction.[8] In a non-randomised comparison, Lard et al.[9] compared the radiographic benefits of treatment with chloroquine or sulphasalazine within 15 days of diagnosis or 123 days after diagnosis in a cohort of over 200 rheumatoid arthritis patients with a symptom duration of just a few months. Over a 2-year period, the median progression in Sharp score was 10 points in the delayed treatment group, as compared with 3.5 points in the early treatment group. In another observational study, the traditional pyramidal approach to therapy comprising sequential initiation of NSAIDs with subsequent DMARD therapy was compared with immediate initiation of DMARD therapy.[10] Once again, this study demonstrated reduced radiographic progression in the early DMARD intervention group. Another observational study, from the Norfolk Arthritis Register in the UK, indicated that the 5-year radiographic outcome was improved in those patients in whom DMARD therapy was initiated within 6 months of the diagnosis of rheumatoid arthritis, as contrasted with those in whom therapy commenced 6 months after the initial diagnosis.

Optimising suppression of synovitis in early rheumatoid arthritis

DMARD and steroid therapy

The understanding that improved outcomes in rheumatoid arthritis are linked to early suppression of synovitis led to another question, namely, whether superior outcomes could be achieved when synovitis is suppressed as completely as possible. A study of such an 'intensive' approach to treatment strategy was undertaken in The Netherlands. This was the COmbinatie therapie Bij Reumatoide Artritis (COBRA) trial that compared sulphasalazine as a monotherapy with a schedule comprising combination sulphasalazine and methotrexate DMARD therapy, in addition to a short course of high-dose prednisolone.[11] In this study, the cumulative inflammatory activity over 1 year was found to be lower in the combination therapy group; furthermore, this was associated with reduced radiographic joint damage, as compared with the monotherapy group.

Despite differences between the groups in terms of cumulative inflammation, the number of swollen and tender joints was not significantly different between treatment groups at the 1-year time point, which is likely to reflect the short-term use of step-down steroid therapy in the combination group, as well as the short-term use of low-dose methotrexate. Participating patients in this cohort were followed up in subsequent years. An interesting finding to emerge from this observation at 5 years was that the radiographic distinction between the two treatment strategies observed at 1 year was still present 5 years later. These findings suggested that an early intensive suppression of synovitis might be responsible for a more enduring retardation in the rate of structural damage to joints.

In the Finnish rheumatoid arthritis combination therapy (FIN-RACo) study, 195 patients with recent onset rheumatoid arthritis in the active phase of disease were randomised to treatment with either a combination of DMARDs and prednisolone, or to a single DMARD, with or without prednisolone.[12] At the end to 2 years, progression in radiographic damage was significantly less in the combination therapy group than in the sulphasalazine monotherapy group. Further subanalyses indicated that for the monotherapy group, a treatment delay of greater than 4 months after disease diagnosis resulted in a significantly reduced rate of remission.

As in the case of the COBRA study, the FIN-RACo cohort have been monitored over time, with the finding that early and aggressive combination therapy gives better results than conventional monotherapy with respect to symptoms and signs, 5-year radiographic progression, and importantly, the incidence of work disability.[13]

The hypothesis that the best patient outcomes can be achieved by suppressing the inflammatory component of disease as optimally as possible with conventional DMARD therapy was tested in the TIght COntrol for Rheumatoid Arthritis (TICORA) trial, in which routine out-patient care was compared with a strategy of individualised intensive out-patient management, using a step-up combination therapy regimen, together with intra-articular and/or intramuscular triamsinolone, as determined by the patient's disease activity score assessed at monthly review.[14] The proportion of patients achieving a good EULAR response was significantly higher in the intensive therapy group than in the routine care group. Similarly, remission rates were highly significantly greater in the intensive therapy group at 65% versus 16% in the routine care group. Similarly, radiographic outcomes were superior in the intensive therapy group than in the standard therapy group. Nonetheless, there was still radiographic

progression over four Sharp points in the intensive therapy group (Fig. 8.2).

Biologicals targeting TNF-α in the treatment of early rheumatoid arthritis

The effects of TNF blockade, with or without concomitant methotrexate therapy, have been compared with methotrexate alone in the early phase of rheumatoid arthritis. The findings of these studies indicate that biological therapies targeting TNF-α have greatest efficacy for improvement in symptoms and signs of disease, as well as prevention of structural damage, when used in combination with methotrexate. Furthermore, this apparent synergy can be achieved with modest methotrexate doses.[15] Clinical experience in the use of anti-TNF drugs confirms these findings. For example, in a study comparing etanercept at a dose of 25 mg twice weekly with methotrexate at a dose of 20 mg once weekly, there was no statistically significant difference in the proportion of patients achieving an ACR 20 response at 1 year, at 69% and 64%, respectively.[16] However, there were significant differences between the two groups at the end of 2 years, at 72% of the etanercept-treated patients achieving an ACR 20 response, versus 59% of the patients treated with methotrexate.[17] In this study, at 2 years

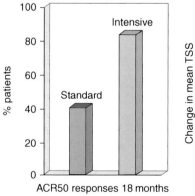
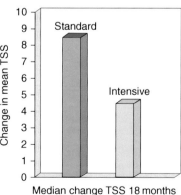

Figure 8.2
TICORA study ACR 50 responses at 12 months and progression of structural damage assessed by the vDH Sharp Score over 18 months.[14]

51% of the patients taking methotrexate alone had no progression in total Sharp score, whereas 63% of the patients on etanercept monotherapy had no progression in total Sharp score. These differences were statistically significant.

In the PREMIER trial, methotrexate-naive patients with early rheumatoid arthritis of less than 3 years' symptom duration were randomised to one of three treatment groups, comprising adalimumab 40 mg every other week together with placebo tablets, methotrexate once weekly rapidly escalated to a dose of 20 mg, together with placebo injections, or adalimumab 40 mg every other week together with methotrexate once weekly, rapidly escalated to a dose of 20 mg. A total of 799 patients were randomised. At week 52, a proportion of patients achieving an ACR 50 response were similar in both the adalimumab monotherapy and methotrexate monotherapy groups, at 42% and 46%, respectively. However, a significantly greater proportion of patients achieved ACR 50 responses with the combination of adalimumab and methotrexate at 62%. Remission criteria defined by a DAS 28 of less than 2.6 was achieved by 43% of patients in the combination therapy arm, versus 23% with adalimumab monotherapy and 21% with methotrexate monotherapy. There was also a significantly better radiographic outcome at 1 year for the group receiving combination therapy as compared with either methotrexate or adalimumab as monotherapy; the change from baseline in total Sharp score was 1.3 in the combination group, 3 in the adalimumab group, and 5.7 in the methotrexate monotherapy group. In contrast to ACR 50 responses, the radiographic outcome was superior with adalimumab alone compared to methotrexate as a monotherapy.[15]

Practice point

Biological therapies targeting TNF-α have greatest efficacy for improvement in symptoms and signs and prevention of structural damage when used in combination with methotrexate

---

Similarly, in the ASPIRE study, methotrexate-naive patients with early rheumatoid arthritis randomised to one of three treatment groups: methotrexate once weekly, rapidly escalated to a dose of 20 mg, together with placebo infusions; methotrexate once weekly, escalated to a dose of 20 mg, together with a dose of infliximab infusions at 3 mg/kg; or methotrexate once weekly, rapidly escalated to a dose of 20 mg with infliximab infusions at 6 mg/kg.[18] At 1 year, a higher proportion of patients achieved ACR 20, 50, and 70 responses in the infliximab and methotrexate combination groups compared with methotrexate alone. For example, 21% of patients on methotrexate alone achieved an ACR 70 response, 33% of patients receiving infliximab at 3 mg/kg together with methotrexate, and 37% of patients receiving 6 mg/kg of infliximab together with methotrexate. Remission criteria at 1 year, as defined by a DAS 28 of less than 2.6, was achieved by 15% of patients on methotrexate monotherapy, 21% of patients receiving infliximab at 3 mg/kg, together with methotrexate, and 31% of patients receiving infliximab at 6 mg/kg together with methotrexate. At 1 year, the median change from baseline in Sharp score for methotrexate monotherapy was 0.43, whereas there was no median progression in infliximab-treated patients at both doses. It is important to point out that about 60% of patients with methotrexate as monotherapy are well controlled, with little or no progression of structural damage. However, at least 25% continue to progress whereas, in this study, infliximab prevented progression in the majority of patients at both dosing regimens.

Collectively, the findings of studies employing TNF blockade in the early phase of rheumatoid arthritis suggests that an advantage of the use of biological therapies targeting TNF over optimised DMARD regimens designed to achieve tight control may be that of superior joint protection.

Comparison of DMARD and biological strategies in early phase rheumatoid arthritis

With the growing appreciation that conventional DMARDs can be used more effectively by intervening early and optimising the dose, it is natural to ask how treatment approaches compare with biological inhibitors of TNF-α. In the future, the same questions will need to be asked of biological therapies targeting other relevant disease molecules. A recent remarkable Dutch multicentre study has compared treatment strategies designed to suppress synovitis in early onset rheumatoid arthritis optimally. The BeSt study (a Dutch acronym for Behandel-Strategieen or treatment strategies) is a single-blind, multicentre, randomised, clinical trial comparing four different treatment strategies:

- sequential substitution monotherapy (treatment group one)

- step-up add-on combination therapy (treatment group two)

- initial combination therapy with a short course of high-dose prednisolone (as employed in the COBRA study) (treatment group three)

- initial combination therapy with the TNF inhibitor infliximab and methotrexate (treatment group four).

The treatment goal for each of these strategies was to obtain a low-level of disease activity of clinical relevance as determined by the DAS 44 score of ≤ 2.4.[19] In order to achieve this goal, patients were monitored intensively every 3 months, and the pharmacological therapy was adjusted by a pre-set algorithm to a more intensive regimen if intervention up to that point had failed to achieve the target DAS 44 of ≤ 2.4. Alternatively, if a patient achieved an adequate response at this level for 6 consecutive months, regardless of which of the four strategic arms was being applied, drugs were subsequently tapered in a predetermined manner to a maintenance dose of monotherapy. Prednisolone and infliximab were always the

first drugs to be taken to zero. In the event of a disease flare following a drug taper, that drug was re-introduced at the last effective dose. Prednisolone could only be re-introduced once.

A total of 508 patients entered the study. The median symptom duration was 23 weeks, and yet this was a cohort with severe disease and 72% had radiographic erosions at baseline. The two combination therapy groups (three and four) achieved a sustained low level of disease activity and functional improvement more rapidly than the groups receiving sequential monotherapy or step-up combination therapy (groups one and two). At 1 year of follow-up, patients treated with both initial combinations (groups three and four) had less radiographic progression than the groups receiving sequential monotherapy (group one) or step-up combination therapy (group two). There was a trend towards less radiographic progression in the infliximab or methotrexate group (group four) over the COBRA regimen group (group three). In a subanalysis of the patients without erosive disease at baseline, there was a statistically significant difference in the rate of radiographic progression favouring patients receiving initial treatment with infliximab and methotrexate, as compared to the strategy starting with the COBRA regimen (group three).

In fact, in this strategy comparison study, there was marked improvement in all groups at the end of 1 year and this is likely to illustrate the value of a tight control approach to suppression of synovitis. For example, over 40% of patients in groups one and two, treated with methotrexate alone, achieved the target suppression of disease activity. It is also of note that patients in the initial combination therapy groups had more rapid relief of symptoms and functional improvement. After the first year of follow-up, 32% of all patients had clinical remission of their disease.

Of interest, further data on the BeSt trial presented at international meetings indicate that of 120 patients receiving initial treatment with infliximab and methotrexate, 77 were responders and able to discontinue infliximab according to protocol. Many of these patients had to recommence infliximab therapy, but 67 of 120 were able to maintain a biological-free remission. These preliminary data raise the possibility that very early intervention with a biological TNF inhibitor, in this case infliximab, might allow induction of biological-free remission. Another small study also supports this hypothesis.[20]

In this study, 20 patients with active early rheumatoid arthritis and mean symptom duration of 6 months were randomised to receive either infliximab at 3 mg/kg or placebo infusions at standard dosing intervals. Four patients began methotrexate at baseline with dose escalation according to a standardised protocol.[20] The first 54 weeks of the study were carried out in a double-blind manner and then infusions were discontinued. Patients were subsequently followed in an observational study and persistent non-responders treated with step-up combination therapy according to a clinic protocol in an open-label manner. Patients treated with infliximab and methotrexate demonstrated a significant reduction in the DAS 28 score at 14, 54, and 104 weeks. At 54 weeks, the median DAS 28 score reflected mild disease (2.84). Remission rates were greater in the patients initially treated with infliximab and methotrexate. Of these, seven patients met ACR remission criteria at some point up to week 104, as compared with two patients in the group taking placebo and methotrexate initially. Median time in remission for the infliximab and methotrexate group was 26 weeks, as compared to 0 weeks in the placebo plus methotrexate group ($P < 0.05$). Following the last infusion of study drug at 46 weeks, patients were observed for a further 58 weeks. Of the 10 patients receiving infliximab in the first year, seven maintained DAS 28 responses, two had an increase in DAS 28 reflecting loss of response, at least 32 weeks after the last infusion, and one failed to respond at any point. Collectively, these data support the concept of a window of opportunity for treatment of early disease and generate the hypothesis that early biological intervention with an anti-TNF agent may allow for induction of subsequent biological-free remission.

In another small study, the ultrasonographic and radiographic effects of immediate or 1-year-delayed addition of infliximab to on-going methotrexate therapy were compared with patients with poor prognosis, erosive early rheumatoid arthritis.[21,22] Twenty-four patients were treated with methotrexate and randomised to receive either infliximab at a dose of 5 mg/kg or placebo infusions. The methotrexate dose was escalated after 18 weeks according to the level of disease activity as indicated by a predetermined protocol. Ultrasonographic measures of inflammation were more rapidly suppressed in the patients receiving early infliximab therapy, and there was a significant difference in vascular signal and synovial thickening between the two groups at 18 weeks. For patients receiving methotrexate alone during the first year, synovial inflammation detected by the ultrasonographic modalities that was still present after 1 year was subsequently suppressed following the addition of infliximab, but by the end of year two, during which all patients received infliximab, there were no significant differences between the two groups with respect to changes from baseline in synovial thickening and vascularity.

From baseline to week 54, there was a median increase of 3.3 in total Sharp score for the infliximab plus methotrexate group, compared with 14 points in the placebo plus methotrexate group ($P = 0.056$). From week 54 through week 110, all patients received infliximab. There was no additional progression in median Sharp score through this time period. This remarkable observation in a small study strongly points to a detrimental impact on joint destruction of delaying anti-TNF treatment in patients with poor-prognosis early rheumatoid arthritis that is active despite optimal treatment with methotrexate.

Conclusions

Much evidence from many studies of rheumatoid arthritis strongly indicate that the magnitude of improvement in symptoms and signs, as well as the rate of reduction in progression of joint destruction, is particularly impressive when drug intervention is initiated at the earliest stages of disease. These observations point to a 'window of opportunity' for optimal disease control and outcome by means of drug intervention and emphasise the importance of early referral to a rheumatologist in cases of suspected rheumatoid arthritis.

References

1. Devlin J, Gough A, Huissoon A et al. The acute phase and function in early rheumatoid arthritis. C-reactive protein levels correlate with functional outcome. J Rheumatol 1997; **24**: 9–13.

2. Gough AK, Lilley J, Eyre S, Holder RL, Emery P. Generalised bone loss in patients with early rheumatoid arthritis. Lancet 1994; **344**: 23–7.

3. Hannonen P, Mottonen T, Hakola M, Oka M. Sulphasalazine in early rheumatoid arthritis. A 48-week double-blind, prospective, placebo-controlled study. Arthritis Rheum 1993; **36**: 1501–9.

4. McGonagle D, Conaghan PG, O'Connor P et al. The relationship between synovitis and bone changes in early untreated rheumatoid arthritis: a controlled magnetic resonance imaging study. Arthritis Rheum 1999; **42**: 1706–11.

5. McQueen FM, Stewart N, Crabbe J et al. Magnetic resonance imaging of the wrist in early rheumatoid arthritis reveals a high prevalence of erosions at four months after symptom onset. Ann Rheum Dis 1998; **57**: 350–6.

6. van der Heijde DM, van Leeuwen MA, van Riel PL, van de Putte LB. Radiographic progression on radiographs of hands and feet during the first 3 years of rheumatoid arthritis measured according to Sharp's method (van der Heijde modification). J Rheumatol 1995; **22**: 1792–6.

7. Egsmose C, Lund B, Borg G et al. Patients with rheumatoid arthritis benefit from early 2nd line therapy: 5 year follow up of a prospective double blind placebo controlled study. J Rheumatol 1995; **22**: 2208–13.

8. van der Heide A, Jacobs JW, Bijlsma JW et al. The effectiveness of early treatment with 'second-line' antirheumatic drugs. A randomized, controlled trial. Ann Intern Med 1996; **124**: 699–707.

9. Lard LR, Visser H, Speyer I et al. Early versus delayed treatment in patients with recent-onset rheumatoid arthritis: comparison of two cohorts who received different treatment strategies. Am J Med 2001; **111**: 446–51.

10. van Aken J, Lard LR, le Cessie S, Hazes JM, Breedveld FC, Huizinga TW. Radiological outcome after four years of early versus delayed treatment strategy in patients with recent onset rheumatoid arthritis. Ann Rheum Dis 2004; **63**: 274–9.

11. Boers M, Verhoeven AC, Markusse HM et al. Randomised comparison of combined step-down prednisolone, methotrexate and sulphasalazine with sulphasalazine alone in early rheumatoid arthritis. Lancet 1997; **350**: 309–18. Erratum in: Lancet 1998; **351**: 220.

12. Mottonen T, Hannonen P, Leirisalo-Repo M et al. Comparison of combination therapy with single-drug therapy in early rheumatoid arthritis: a randomised trial. FIN-RACo trial group. Lancet 1999; **353**: 1568–73.

13. Puolakka K, Kautiainen H, Mottonen T et al. and FIN-RACo Trial Group. Early suppression of disease activity is essential for maintenance of work capacity in patients with recent-onset rheumatoid arthritis: five-year experience from the FIN-RACo trial. Arthritis Rheum 2005; **52**: 36–41.

14. Grigor C, Capell H, Stirling A et al. Effect of a treatment strategy of tight control for rheumatoid arthritis (the TICORA study): a single-blind randomised controlled trial. Lancet 2004; **364**: 263–9.

15. Breedveld FC, Weisman MH, Kavanaugh AF et al. The PREMIER study: a multicenter, randomized, double-blind clinical trial of combination therapy with adalimumab plus methotrexate versus methotrexate alone or adalimumab alone in patients with early, aggressive rheumatoid arthritis who had not had previous methotrexate treatment. Arthritis Rheum 2006; **54**: 26–37.

16. Bathon JM, Martin RW, Fleischmann RM et al. A comparison of etanercept and methotrexate in patients with early rheumatoid arthritis. N Engl J Med 2000; **343**: 1586–93. Erratum in: N Engl J Med 2001; **344**: 240. N Engl J Med 2001; **344**: 76.

17. Genovese MC, Bathon JM, Martin RW et al. Etanercept versus methotrexate in patients with early rheumatoid arthritis: two-year radiographic and clinical outcomes. Arthritis Rheum 2002; **46**: 1443–50.

18. St Clair EW, van der Heijde DM, Smolen JS et al. and Active-Controlled Study of Patients Receiving Infliximab for the Treatment of Rheumatoid Arthritis of Early Onset Study Group. Combination of infliximab and methotrexate therapy for early rheumatoid arthritis: a randomized, controlled trial. Arthritis Rheum 2004; **50**: 3432–43.

19. Goekoop-Ruiterman YP, de Vries-Bouwstra JK, Allaart CF *et al.* Clinical and radiographic outcomes of four different treatment strategies in patients with early rheumatoid arthritis (the BeSt study): a randomized, controlled trial. *Arthritis Rheum* 2005; **52**: 3381–90.

20. Quinn MA, Conaghan PG, O'Connor PJ *et al.* Very early treatment with infliximab in addition to methotrexate in early, poor-prognosis rheumatoid arthritis reduces magnetic resonance imaging evidence of synovitis and damage, with sustained benefit after infliximab withdrawal: results from a twelve-month randomized, double-blind, placebo-controlled trial. *Arthritis Rheum* 2005; **52**: 27–35.

21. Taylor PC, Steuer A, Gruber J *et al.* Comparison of ultrasonographic assessment of synovitis and joint vascularity with radiographic evaluation in a randomized, placebo-controlled study of infliximab therapy in early rheumatoid arthritis. *Arthritis Rheum* 2004; **50**: 1107–16.

22. Taylor PC, Steuer A, Gruber J *et al.* Ultrasonographic and radiographic results from a two-year controlled trial of immediate or one-year-delayed addition of infliximab to ongoing methotrexate therapy in patients with erosive early rheumatoid arthritis. *Arthritis Rheum* 2006; **54**: 47–53.

23. Sharp JT, Wolfe F, Mitchell DM, Bloch DA. The progression of erosion and joint space narrowing scores in rheumatoid arthritis during the first twenty-five years of disease. *Arthritis Rheum* 1991; **34**: 660–8.

9 Emerging biological therapies

B-cell targeted therapy
Modulation of co-stimulation
Biological therapies in clinical development
Future therapies

Despite the advances in pharmacological intervention in the management of rheumatoid arthritis, including the more effective use of traditional DMARDs and the advent of biological TNF inhibitors, there is still unmet need. A proportion of patients remain refractory to conventional treatment and anti-TNF agents and among those who respond, not all achieve clinical remission. Furthermore, all the available therapies are associated with some degree of toxicity and currently available anti-TNF therapies are exceedingly costly. The marked success of the development of TNF inhibitors, together with the recognition that there remains considerable unmet need, has led to a drive to develop biological therapies targeting other relevant disease molecules. Some are in the early stages of clinical development, such as alternative inhibitors of IL-1 to IL-1 receptor antagonist, discussed in the last chapter, and inhibitors of pro-inflammatory cytokines such as IL-6 and IL-15. There are two other biological agents at an advanced stage of development, one of which targets B cells and the other a co-stimulatory molecule.

B-cell targeted therapy

The role of B cells in the pathogenesis of rheumatoid arthritis is not fully understood. Nonetheless, there are a number of known B lymphocyte functions which are of potential importance, including their role in antigen presentation, secretion of pro-inflammatory cytokines, production of rheumatoid factor and thus their role in immune complex formation, and co-stimulation of T cells. Immune complexes are one trigger to production of TNF and other pro-inflammatory cytokines. B cells are also implicated in the process of ectopic lymphoid organogenesis in the rheumatoid synovium.

CD20 antigen

The CD20 antigen is highly expressed on B cells but not on stem, dendritic, or plasma cells (Fig. 9.1). The CD20 antigen is expressed on a range of pre-B cells, immature B cells, activated cells, and memory cells. CD20+ B cells represent a prominent population in the rheumatoid synovial tissue in the majority of patients. The chimeric mouse–human monoclonal antibody directed against CD20, rituximab, binds to the extracellular domain of the CD20 antigen. It initiates complement-mediated B-cell lysis and may permit antibody-dependent, cell-mediated cytotoxicity when the Fc portion of the antibody is recognised by corresponding receptors on cytotoxic cells. Rituximab may also initiate apoptosis and also the ability of B cells to respond to antigen or other stimuli.[1] Rituximab initially found a role in the clinic as a single-agent treatment for relapsed or refractory low-grade or follicular CD20+ B-cell non-Hodgkin's lymphoma, for which it was approved. There was, therefore, a wide experience of rituximab in haematological oncology prior to clinical trials of this drug in rheumatoid arthritis, and its recent licence granted for TNF inhibitor-refractory patients.

The efficacy of rituximab in active rheumatoid arthritis was tested in 161 patients who had failed to respond adequately to treatment with methotrexate at a dose of at least 10 mg once weekly for at least 16 weeks. Patients were assigned to one of four treatment regimens: (i) intravenous rituximab alone in the form of a 1 g infusion on days 1 and 15; (ii) methotrexate alone as a comparator arm; (iii) intravenous

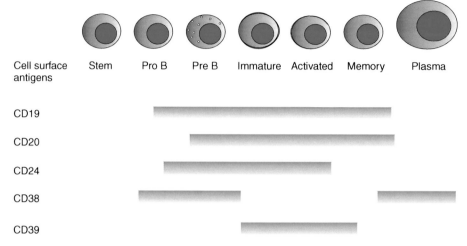

Figure 9.1
Expression of the CD20 antigen during maturation of B cells.

rituximab with cyclophosphamide infusions at a dose of 750 mg on days 3 and 17; or (iv) rituximab and methotrexate. All patients received 100 mg methylprednisolone just before each treatment (or intravenous placebo), in addition to prednisolone 60 mg daily on day 2 and days 4–7 and 30 mg daily on days 8–14. The primary end-point was the proportion of patients achieving an ACR 50 response at week 24, and exploratory analyses were undertaken at week 48.[2] At week 24, a significantly greater proportion of patients achieved an ACR 50 in the rituximab and methotrexate combination group (43%; $P = 0.005$), and the rituximab and cyclophosphamide combination group (41%; $P = 0.005$) than in the group receiving methotrexate as monotherapy (13%). Of the patients receiving rituximab alone, 33% achieved an ACR 50 response, but this failed to reach statistical significance as compared with methotrexate alone ($P = 0.059$). In all the rituximab groups, the mean change from baseline in disease activity score was significant as compared with methotrexate alone.

At 48 weeks, an exploratory analysis of the ACR responses in the rituximab and methotrexate group demonstrated 35% of patients responding at the ACR 50 level, and 15% of the ACR 70 level, significantly greater than the 5% and 0% responses at ACR 50 and ACR 70 levels, respectively, in the methotrexate group. In the rituximab and cyclophosphamide treatment arm, 27% of patients achieved an ACR 50 response.

Rituximab treatment was associated with near-complete peripheral blood B-cell depletion, persisting throughout the 24-week period of the primary analysis. Patients in the rituximab groups were noted to have a substantial and rapid reduction in the concentration of rheumatoid factor levels in serum, but despite peripheral B cell depletion, immunoglobulin levels did not change substantially.[2]

Surprisingly, in view of the profound peripheral B-cell depletion, the overall incidence of infection reported was similar in the control and rituximab groups, at 24 and 48 weeks. By week 24, four patients in the rituximab groups had suffered a serious infection and one in the control group. Two further serious infections were reported during the extended 48-week period in the rituximab groups, one of which was fatal. Infusion reactions were reported in 36% of patients receiving rituximab and 30% of patients receiving placebo, although most were characterised as mild or moderate. Infusion reactions included hypotension, hypertension, flushing, pruritis, and rash. These features are thought to be caused by a cytokine release syndrome associated with marked cell lysis.

Preliminary results of a phase III trial of rituximab in active rheumatoid arthritis were presented at the 2005 European League Against Rheumatism meeting.[3] A total of 465 patients with active disease were recruited. They had to have failed at least one DMARD other than methotrexate and to have been treated with methotrexate as a single DMARD for at least 12 weeks, with 4 weeks of stable therapy at a dose of at least 10 mg once weekly. All other DMARDs were withdrawn at least 4 weeks prior to randomisation and 8 weeks for infliximab, adalimumab, or leflunomide. Patients were randomised to receive either placebo infusions or rituximab at a dose of 50 mg or 1 g on days 1 and 15, together with one of three glucocorticoid options, comprising glucocorticoid placebo, 100 mg of intravenous methylprednisolone prior to each rituximab infusion, or 100 mg of methylprednisolone prior to each infusion in addition to oral corticosteroid. The results at 24 weeks confirmed the significant efficacy of a single course of rituximab in active rheumatoid arthritis when combined with continuing methotrexate. This benefit was independent of glucocorticoids, although methylprednisolone on day 1 reduced the incidence and severity of first rituximab infusion reactions by about one-third. Both rituximab doses were efficacious, with the higher dose of 1 g 2 weeks apart showing a trend towards higher ACR 70 and EULAR good responses. Adverse events reported up to 24 weeks were largely infusion-related, particularly at the time of the first infusion.

Conclusions

Recent advances in the understanding of the pathogenesis of rheumatoid arthritis emphasise the critical role played by peripheral blood B cells in self-sustaining chronic inflammatory processes. The available data suggest that rituximab is most effective in a proportion of rheumatoid factor positive patients and that this drug will be a promising addition to the therapeutic armamentarium for the treatment of rheumatoid arthritis. It is likely that its major use in clinical practice will be confined to the TNF inhibitor-refractory population in the short term, until there is broader experience and confidence regarding potential adverse effects. At the present time, there are uncertainties regarding the implications of long-term peripheral B cell depletion and the timing and need for re-dosing with rituximab in patients who respond. Current research suggests that restoration of peripheral B cell numbers takes 6–18 months after depletion therapy, and further studies are needed to identify the optimum regimens that can be used for maintenance therapy that will provide efficacy and limit toxicity. Although there is already a substantial body of data regarding the safety profile of rituximab for treatment of non-Hodgkin's lymphoma, some of the associated adverse events are related to circulating tumour loads. Low infection rates have been reported in oncology, and this is re-assuring with regard to the rheumatoid population, although close monitoring of immunocompetence and for the occurrence of opportunistic infections in rheumatoid patients exposed to rituximab is advisable.

Other experimental biological therapies targeting B cells

Alternative strategies to target the B-cell compartment include the use of antibodies to B lymphocyte stimulator or BlyS (Fig. 9.2). BLyS is a naturally occurring protein required for the development of B-lymphocytes into mature plasma cells. Elevated levels of BLyS in rheumatoid arthritis are believed to contribute to the production of autoantibodies. Belimumab, or LymphoStat-B, is a human anti-BLyS monoclonal antibody currently in clinical development for the treatment of rheumatoid arthritis and other rheumatic indications. An alternative approach to BLyS inhibition in early

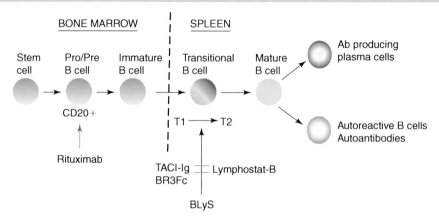

Figure 9.2
Targeting B cells in rheumatoid arthritis.

stages of clinical development is to block signalling through BLyS receptors using a soluble receptor such as transmembrane activator and calcium modulator and cyclophilin ligand interactor immunoglobulin (TACI-Ig). Preliminary results of a phase II double-blind placebo-controlled study of belimumab in active rheumatoid arthritis were presented at the American College of Rheumatology meeting in the autumn of 2005. A total of 283 patients were enrolled with active rheumatoid arthritis despite prior treatment with non-biological and/or biological DMARDs. Biological DMARDs had to be washed out prior to enrolment. Patients were randomised to receive intravenous belimumab at a dose of 1, 4, or 10 mg/kg or placebo infusions on days 0, 14, and 28, then every 28 days through 24 weeks. The ACR 20 response at week 24 in the combined belimumab groups was 29% compared to 16% in the placebo group, with no dose response observed. The antibody was well tolerated.[4]

These preliminary findings with a functional inhibitor of B cells are surprising, given the effectiveness of rituximab, a B-cell depleter, in the treatment of rheumatoid arthritis. This may simply represent a pharmacokinetic problem and that too low a dose of belimumab was

used. An alternative explanation might be that the effectiveness of rituximab is not directly related to its effects on B cells.

Modulation of co-stimulation

Co-stimulation is an essential step in the induction of adaptive immune responses. Although the role of T cells in the perpetuation of rheumatoid arthritis has been debated and remains poorly understood, it has long been believed that T-cell activation is a key event in the pathogenesis. Successful T-cell activation requires multiple signals. One signal is provided by presentation of an antigen bound to cell-surface MHC molecules on antigen-presenting cells to a specific T-cell receptor. In the absence of further signals, T cells become unresponsive and may ultimately be eliminated through apoptosis. An important co-stimulatory signal is provided by an interaction between members of the B-7 family (either CD80 or CD86) on antigen-presenting cells and CD28 on T cells. Other key interactions between antigen-presenting cells and T cells are mediated by binding of ICAM-1 to LFA-1, CD40 to CD40 ligand, LFA-3 to CD2, and so on. After activation, T cells express CTLA-4 which interferes with the B-7–CD-28 interaction and helps to return the cells to the quiescent state.

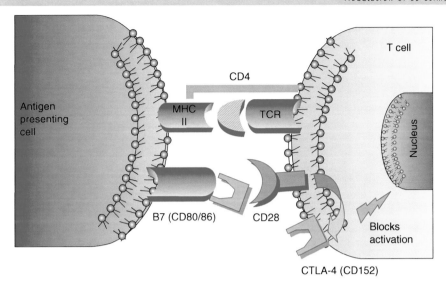

Figure 9.3

Successful T-cell activation requires multiple signals. One signal is provided by presentation of an antigen bound to cell surface MHC molecules on antigen-presenting cells to a specific T cell receptor. In the absence of further signals, T cells become unresponsive and may ultimately be eliminated through apoptosis. An important co-stimulatory signal is provided by an interaction between members of the B-7 family (either CD80 or CD86) on antigen-presenting cells and CD28 on T cells. After activation, T cells express CTLA-4 which interferes with the B-7–CD-28 interaction and helps to return the cells to the quiescent state.

Abatacept is a novel, fully human fusion protein, comprising the extracellular portion of CTLA-4 and the Fc fragment of a human IgG_1; it is the first biological co-stimulatory modulator to be in advanced clinical trials. Abatacept binds to CD80 and CD86 on antigen-presenting cells, thus preventing these molecules from binding their ligand, CD28, on T cells, with consequent inhibition of optimal T-cell activation. *In vitro*, abatacept decreases T-cell proliferation and inhibits production of TNF-α, IFN-γ, and IL-2.

Clinical data

In December 2005, abatacept (orencia) was approved by the US FDA for the treatment of patients with rheumatoid arthritis who have had an inadequate response to other drugs. Abatacept has been evaluated in five randomised, double-blind, placebo-controlled trials in adults with active rheumatoid arthritis

with an inadequate response to conventional DMARDs such as methotrexate or to TNF inhibitors.

Following initial pilot studies that demonstrated efficacy of etanercept in treating the signs and symptoms of rheumatoid arthritis,[5] the findings were confirmed in a multicentre phase II study of 339 patients with active rheumatoid arthritis despite methotrexate treatment.[6] In this study, patients were randomised to receive infusions of either placebo, abatacept at a dose of 2 mg/kg or 10 mg/kg at baseline, 2 weeks, 4 weeks, and then monthly through to 6 months. ACR 20% responses were achieved in 60%, 41.9%, and 35.3% of patients receiving abatacept at 10 mg/kg, 2 mg/kg, or placebo infusions, respectively. At the more stringent ACR 50% response level, the figures were 36.5%, 22.9%, and 11.8%. Improvements in the individual components of the ACR response criteria were generally greater in the 10 mg/kg group than the 2 mg/kg group. No deaths, malignancies, or opportunistic infections were reported for any patient receiving abatacept during the 6 months of therapy. Patients in the phase II study continued on blinded therapy for an additional 6 months, during which time response to therapy was maintained. For patients receiving abatacept at 10 mg/kg, the ACR 70, ACR 50, and ACR 20 response rates were 21%, 42%, and 63%, respectively, compared with 8%, 20%, and 36%, respectively, for patients receiving placebo infusions.

Preliminary data have been presented from a large phase III study of abatacept in methotrexate-refractory patients and the findings of a second phase III study of abatacept therapy in RA patients with an inadequate response to TNF antagonist therapy have recently been reported.[7] In the first of these studies (the AIM study), 652 patients with an inadequate response to methotrexate were randomly assigned to receive either placebo or a fixed dose of abatacept approximating 10 mg/kg, while remaining on background methotrexate therapy.[8] Patients receiving abatacept showed greater improvement in all ACR response criteria through 12 months than placebo-treated patients. Furthermore, patients on the abatacept and methotrexate combination also showed slowing of the progression of structural damage at 1.2 total Sharp score points over 1 year, compared with methotrexate alone, where the rate of progression was 2.3 Sharp score points.[9]

In the second Phase III study (ATTAIN; Abatacept Trial in Treatment of INadequate Responders), abatacept therapy was evaluated in 391 patients who failed to respond adequately to at least 3 months of therapy with a TNF inhibitor (Fig. 9.4).[7] Patients were randomly assigned to receive either placebo or the same fixed dose of abatacept approximating 10 mg/kg. Anti-TNF therapy was discontinued at the time of enrolment if it had not been

done previously. Patients receiving abatacept showed greater improvement in all ACR response criteria through 6 months than placebo-treated patients. Furthermore, a DAS 28 remission was achieved in 10% of patients receiving abatacept versus only 1% of patients receiving placebo infusions plus DMARDs. ACR 20 responses were seen irrespective of whether the patients had been exposed to prior etanercept or infliximab treatment or both anti-TNF therapies without adequate response. Improvement in physical function was also significantly increased in the abatacept group (47% versus 23%). The incidence of infection was slightly higher in the abatacept group than in the placebo group, although no specific infection was clearly more frequent, and the intensity of infections appeared similar in the two groups. There were no significant differences in the numbers of patients discontinuing treatment as a result of infection or in the incidence of serious infections.

Abatacept may be used as monotherapy or concomitantly with DMARDs other than TNF antagonists. It is not recommended for use concomitantly with IL-1 antagonists. The encouraging clinical trial data indicate that abatacept, like rituximab, represents a new addition to the therapeutic armamentarium for patients with rheumatoid arthritis who have not responded adequately to TNF blockade. As yet, however, the comparative effects of abatacept, rituximab, and TNF blockade on structural damage are unknown. It is clear that where clinical responses are unsatisfactory, combination therapy with methotrexate and an anti-TNF agent may still confer significant joint protection compared with methotrexate alone. Thus the merits of switching a patient from an anti-TNF inhibitor to abatacept or rituximab on the basis of an inadequate clinical response are not yet clear-cut with respect to disease modification. Other factors likely to determine the future uptake and relative positioning of new biologicals in the clinic include further long-term safety data, comparative cost-effectiveness analyses, and the perceived convenience of intravenous administration.

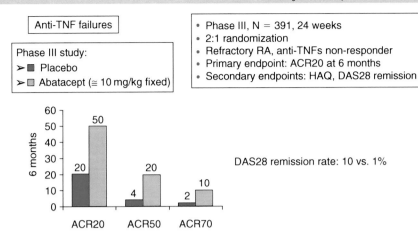

Figure 9.4
Clinical responses observed in the ATTAIN study of abatacept in a TNF inhibitor-refractory population. Modified from Genovese et al.[7] with permission.

Biological therapies in clinical development

Based on *in vitro* diseased tissue and pre-clinical animal model studies, several other inflammatory cytokines have been identified as potential therapeutic targets in rheumatoid arthritis. Two particularly promising targets are IL-6 and IL-15.

IL-6 blockade

IL-6 is another pleiotropic cytokine abundantly expressed in rheumatoid synovium and detectable in the peripheral blood of rheumatoid patients during active phases of the disease. IL-6 binds soluble and membrane-bound receptors and their interaction with a gp130 molecule transduces intracellular signalling with mediation of gene activation and a wide range of biological activities. These include B-cell differentiation into immunoglobulin-secreting plasma cells, T-cell activation, and platelet production. IL-6 also regulates the production of acute phase proteins by hepatocytes and activates osteoclasts to absorb bone. Mice lacking the IL-6 gene are protected from arthritis induction.[10]

Transitory, clinical improvements were reported in a small, uncontrolled group of patients with active rheumatoid arthritis following 10 consecutive days of once-daily intravenous murine monoclonal anti-IL-6 antibody.[11] These improvements were accompanied by a fall in serum C-reactive protein concentrations.

An alternative approach to blocking the bioactivity of IL-6 is to use antibodies to the IL-6 receptor. Tocilizumab (previously known as MRA) is an anti-human IL-6 receptor antibody of IgG-1 subclass. The antibody has been humanised by grafting the complementarity-determining regions of a murine anti-human IL-6 receptor monoclonal antibody onto human IgG_1. Tocilizumab competes for both the membrane-bound and soluble forms of human IL-6 receptor, so inhibiting the biological activity of IL-6.

In a multicentre, Japanese, double-blind, placebo-controlled trial, 164 patients with refractory rheumatoid arthritis were randomised to receive either placebo infusions or MRA at a dose of 4 mg/kg or 8 mg/kg. The antibody and placebo were administered intravenously every 4 weeks for a total of 3 months. IL-6 receptor blockade reduced disease activity in a dose-dependent manner. At 3 months, ACR 20 responses were reported in 78% of patients receiving MRA at 8 mg/kg, 57% of those in the 4 mg/kg group, and 11% in the placebo group. ACR 50 responses were seen in 40% of patients in the 8 mg/kg MRA group and only 1.9% in the placebo group. In this Japanese study, the overall incidence of adverse events was similar in all groups. Mild and transient derangements of liver function tests were noted, as well as reductions in white blood cell counts. A blood cholesterol increase was observed in 44% of the patients but antibodies to MRA were only detected in two patients.

In a European multicentre, randomised, clinical trial, tocilizumab was used either as monotherapy (by discontinuation of methotrexate) or concomitantly with methotrexate therapy and compared with placebo infusions in patients maintained on a fixed dose of methotrexate over 20 weeks (CHARISMA; Chugai Humanized Anti-human Recombinant Interleukin-Six Monoclonal Antibody). A total of 359 patients with established rheumatoid arthritis and an inadequate response to methotrexate were recruited.[12]

In this study, the percentage of patients receiving methotrexate alone achieving ACR 20, 50, and 70% responses was 41%, 29%, and 16%, respectively. Tocilizumab was given at one of three dose regimens – 2 mg/kg, 4 mg/kg, or 8 mg/kg – either as a monotherapy or in combination with methotrexate. As in the Japanese study, a dose–response effect was seen, with the best responses at the highest doses of tocilizumab. As a monotherapy, 8 mg/kg of tocilizumab gave rise to ACR 20, 50, and 70 responses in 63%, 41%, and 16%, respectively. In combination with methotrexate, the corresponding figures were 74%, 53%, and 37%, significantly higher than the methotrexate and placebo infusion group. In general, tocilizumab was well tolerated in the CHARISMA study. Anti-tocilizumab antibodies were observed in the monotherapy groups receiving the two lowest doses of antibody, but none

occurred in the 8 mg/kg group, whether given as monotherapy or in combination. A small proportion of patients who started the study with a normal neutrophil count experienced neutropenia when treated with the higher dose of tocilizumab at 8 mg/kg. Three new cases of serious infection were noted in the combination therapy group receiving 8 mg/kg of tocilizumab but four serious infections were noted in the 2 mg/kg monotherapy group, with none noted in the methotrexate monotherapy group. Four cases of anaphylactic reaction were reported out of 107 patients treated with the two lower doses of tocilizumab as a monotherapy. As in the Japanese study, moderate but reversible increases in mean non-fasting total cholesterol and triglycerides were observed over the study period. However, there was also a rise in HDL cholesterol and the mean atherogenic index was unchanged.

In conclusion, these studies validate IL-6 as a target for therapy in rheumatoid arthritis and a potentially promising means of controlling disease activity. Tocilizumab treatment, either as monotherapy or combination therapy with methotrexate, is well tolerated in the majority of cases, with a safety pattern that is consistent with other biological and immunosuppressive therapies. Further phase III studies are under way to further investigate IL-6 blockade.

IL-15 blockade

IL-15 is another potential therapeutic target of interest across a range of inflammatory pathologies. In rheumatoid arthritis, it is detectable in inflamed joints and serves as a powerful T-cell chemo-attractant. T cells from rheumatoid synovial membranes have the capability to induce TNF-α synthesis by blood- or synovial-derived macrophages through cell membrane contact, and there is evidence that IL-15 is one factor capable of sustaining this activity.[13] Blockade of IL-15 ameliorates animal models of rheumatoid arthritis and IL-15 levels in the rheumatoid synovium correlate with TNF-α activity.

In a phase I/II 12-week, dose-ascending, placebo-controlled, double-blind proof-of-concept study, a fully human IgG$_1$ anti-IL-15 antibody, AMG 714, was tested in 30 rheumatoid arthritis patients. The antibody was administered in dose-ascending order to six cohorts of five patients by single subcutaneous infusion. The patients were followed up for 28 days and, in the absence of dose-limiting toxicity by day 28, all patients received four additional doses of AMG 714 at weekly intervals by open-label extension. The antibody was well tolerated clinically, with no significant effects on T lymphocyte subsets and natural killer cell numbers. Substantial improvements in disease activity were observed, with 63% achieving an ACR 20 response, 38% achieving an ACR 50, and 25% achieving ACR 70.[14]

AMG 714 is being tested in on-going clinical trials, and interim analyses have been presented at the American College of Rheumatology meeting in 2004.[15] Rheumatoid patients with active disease despite treatment with at least one conventional DMARD but naive to biological therapy were randomised to receive placebo or one of four doses of AMG 714 – 40, 80, 160, or 280 mg injected subcutaneously once every 2 weeks. All patients received two loading doses of AMG 714 or placebo, according to treatment allocation. Stable background methotrexate, NSAIDs, and low-dose corticosteroids were continued. Patients were treated over 12 weeks with clinical assessments every 2 weeks for the first 16 weeks. Data were presented for 110 patients, which had been collected over the 14-week period. At 12 weeks, 62% of patients receiving the 280-mg dose achieved an ACR 20% response versus 26% of placebo-treated patients. At 14 weeks, 68% of patients receiving AMG 714 at the 280-mg dose achieved a reduction from baseline in CRP exceeding 20% versus 39% of patients receiving placebo injections. There were no differences in adverse events, infections, or serious adverse events between the groups in this interim analysis.

These preliminary data are promising, but must be interpreted with some caution because of the small numbers studied to this point. However, IL-15 represents a potentially interesting target because of its multifaceted pro-inflammatory role in rheumatoid arthritis. In particular, in addition to its involvement in the pro-inflammatory cascade, IL-15 is required for the maintenance of CD8$^+$ memory T cells. Theoretically, therefore, IL-15 blockade might diminish the inflammatory component of disease and the self-directed T-cell immunological memory that characterises the autoimmune response.[16,17] The full data set from placebo-controlled studies of IL-15 blockade in rheumatoid arthritis is, therefore, awaited with great interest.

Future therapies

The expense and inconvenience of parenteral administration of currently available biological agents is such that development of less expensive, orally active, synthetic agents that inhibit bioactivity of TNF-α or other relevant pro-inflammatory cytokines is an attractive goal. One approach that has generated much interest is to use inhibitors of p38 map kinase to block signalling in the p38 pathway, and thus the post-transcriptional stabilisation of mRNA for the major inflammatory cytokines TNF-α and IL-1, as well as other proteins such as cyclo-oxygenase 2. A number of p38 map kinase inhibitors have been developed, and there is encouraging preliminary pre-clinical data demonstrating amelioration of disease in the established phase of collagen-induced arthritis.[18] The full results of human clinical trials are awaited, although there have been preliminary reports of hepatic and other toxicity with some compounds. Because of toxicity concerns, there is interest in more selective targets for inhibition of inflammatory gene expression, for example, map kinase activated-protein kinase II, a major substrate of p38α and p38β, and downstream post-transcriptional events. Other approaches to inhibition of TNF include oral inhibitors of the enzyme TNF-α-converting enzyme (TACE), which cleaves membrane-bound TNF from the surface of producer cells to yield the soluble form of the cytokine. Similarly, another approach to inhibition of active IL-1β is to use oral inhibitors of caspase-1, thereby preventing the cleavage and release of membrane-bound IL-1β from producer cells. However, it is important to bear in mind that many of the reported adverse events associated with biological agents targeting TNF-α, particularly infective complications, were anticipated given the specificity of the drug for a single target with well-defined biological activities. In contrast, because of their multiple intracellular actions, it may prove much harder to predict the spectrum of toxicities that could arise from administration of small molecules, currently under development, that indirectly target the TNF-α or other cytokine pathways.

References

1. Tsokos GC. B cells, be gone – B-cell depletion in the treatment of rheumatoid arthritis. *N Engl J Med* 2004; **350**: 2546–8.

2. Edwards JC, Szczepanski L, Szechinski J *et al.* Efficacy of B-cell-targeted therapy with rituximab in patients with rheumatoid arthritis. *N Engl J Med* 2004; **350**: 2572–81.

3. Emery P, Filipowicz-Sosnowska A, Szczepanski L *et al.* Primary analysis of a double-blind, placebo-controlled, dose-ranging trial of rituximab, an anti-CD20 monoclonal antibody, in patients with rheumatoid arthritis receiving methotrexate (DANCER trial). *Ann Rheum Dis* 2005; **64 (Suppl 3)**: 182.

4. McKay J, Chwalinska-Sadowska H, Boling E *et al.* Efficacy and safety of belimumab (BMAB), a fully human monoclonal antibody to B lymphocyte stimulator (BLyS) for the treatment of rheumatoid arthritis. *Arthritis Rheum Suppl* 2005; **64 (Suppl 3)**: S710.

5. Moreland LW, Alten R, Van den Bosch F *et al.* Co-stimulatory blockade in patients with rheumatoid arthritis: a pilot, dose-finding, double-blind, placebo-controlled clinical trial evaluating CTLA-4Ig and LEA29Y eighty-five days after the first infusion. *Arthritis Rheum* 2002; **46**: 1470–9.

6. Kremer JM, Westhovens R, Leon M *et al.* Treatment of rheumatoid arthritis by selective inhibition of T-cell activation with fusion protein CTLA4Ig. *N Engl J Med* 2003; **349**: 1907–15.

7. Genovese MC, Becker JC, Schiff M *et al.* Abatacept for rheumatoid arthritis refractory to tumor necrosis factor alpha inhibition. *N Engl J Med* 2005; **353**: 1114–23.

8. Russell A, Kremer J, Westhovens R *et al.* Efficacy and safety of the selective co-stimulation modulator abatacept with methotrexate for treating rheumatoid arthritis: 1-year clinical and radiographic results from the phase III AIM (Abatacept in INadequate responders to Methotrexate) trial. *J Rheumatol* 2005; **32**: 1394.

9. Genant H, Peterfy C, Paira S *et al.* Abatacept significantly inhibits structural damage progression as assessed by the Genant-modified Sharp scoring system in rheumatoid arthritis patients with inadequate methotrexate responses. *Ann Rheum Dis* 2005; **64 (Suppl 3)**: 56.

10. Boe A, Baiocchi M, Carbonatto M, Papoian R, Serlupi-Crescenzi O. Interleukin 6 knock-out mice are resistant to antigen-induced experimental arthritis. *Cytokine* 1999; **11**: 1057–64.

11. Wendling D, Racadot E, Wijdenes J. Treatment of severe rheumatoid arthritis by anti-interleukin 6 monoclonal antibody. *J Rheumatol* 1993; **20**: 259–62.

12. Maini RN, Taylor PC, Szechinski J *et al.* for the CHARISMA Study Group. Randomized clinical trial of the IL-6 receptor antagonist, tocilizumab (MRA) in rheumatoid arthritis patients with an incomplete response to methotrexate in Europe (CHARISMA). *Arthritis Rheum* 2006; In press.

13. Liew FY, McInnes IB. Role of interleukin 15 and interleukin 18 in inflammatory response. *Ann Rheum Dis* 2002; **61 (Suppl 2)**: ii100–2.

14. Baslund B, Tvede N, Danneskiold-Samsoe B *et al.* Targeting interleukin-15 in patients with rheumatoid arthritis: a proof-of-concept study. *Arthritis Rheum* 2005; **52**: 2686–92.

15. McInnes I, Martin R, Zimmerman-Gorska I *et al.* Safety and efficacy of a human monoclonal antibody to IL-15 (AMG 714) in patients with rheumatoid arthritis (RA): results from a multi-center, randomized, double-blind, placebo-controlled trial. *Arthritis Rheum* 2004; **50 (Suppl)**: S241.

16. Zhang X, Sun S, Hwang I, Tough DF, Sprent J. Potent and selective stimulation of memory-phenotype CD8+ T cells *in vivo* by IL-15. *Immunity* 1998; **8**: 591–9.

17. Ku CC, Murakami M, Sakamoto A, Kappler J, Marrack P. Control of homeostasis of CD8+ memory T cells by opposing cytokines. *Science* 2000; **288**: 675–8.

18. Nabozny GH, Souza D, Raymond E, Pargellis C, Regan J. Inhibition of established collagen induced arthritis (CIA) with BIRB 796, a selective inhibitor of p38 map kinase. *Arthritis Rheum* 2001; **44 (Suppl)**: S38.

Index

Page numbers in *italics* refer to information that is shown only in a table or diagram.